Studies in Diplomacy and International Relations

Series Editors
Donna Lee
Keele University
Keele, UK

Marcus Holmes
College of William & Mary
Williamsburg, USA

Founded over two decades ago by Geoff Berridge, the *Studies in Diplomacy and International Relations* (*SDIR*) series aims to publish the best new scholarship interrogating and demonstrating the central role of diplomacy in contemporary international relations. We are proud to continue this tradition by publishing diverse and cutting-edge research from a global community of scholars that investigates diplomatic theory and practice, the diplomacy of sustainability and climate change, trade, economic and business diplomacy, international negotiations, the diplomacy of global health, the constitution and effects of great power politics, global communications, and public diplomacy, among other topics. *SDIR* seeks to publish work that will be of interest to communities of scholars, practitioners of diplomacy, and policymakers alike.

For an informal discussion for a book in the series, please contact one of the series editors Donna Lee (d.lee@keele.ac.uk) or Marcus Holmes (mholmes@wm.edu), or Commissioning Editor Isobel Cowper-Coles (isobel.cowpercoles@palgrave.com).

For the correct version of the proposal form, please contact Isobel Cowper-Coles.

This series is indexed in Scopus.

Humphrey Ngala Ndi • Henry Ngenyam Bang
Zebulon Suifon Takwa • Anna Tasha Mbur
Editors

Health Diplomacy
in Africa

Trends, Challenges, and Perspectives

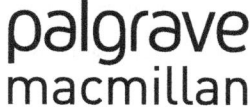

palgrave
macmillan

Editors
Humphrey Ngala Ndi (iD)
High Commission for the Republic of
Cameroon
London, UK

University of Yaounde I
Yaounde, Cameroon

Zebulon Suifon Takwa
United Nations Development
Programme
Harare, Zimbabwe

Henry Ngenyam Bang (iD)
Department of Disaster and
Emergency Management
Coventry University
Coventry, UK

Anna Tasha Mbur
High Commission for the Republic of
Cameroon
London, UK

ISSN 2731-3921   ISSN 2731-393X   (electronic)
Studies in Diplomacy and International Relations
ISBN 978-3-031-41251-6   ISBN 978-3-031-41249-3   (eBook)
https://doi.org/10.1007/978-3-031-41249-3

This Palgrave Macmillan imprint is published by the registered company Springer Nature
Switzerland AG.
The registered company address is: Gewerbestrasse 11, 6330 Cham, Switzerland

Paper in this product is recyclable.

PREFACE

The greatest threat to the survival of post-colonial African governments and states is weak social development, especially health. If Africa must be self-sufficient in its resources and people, it must embrace the spirit of *unbuntu*, a Zulu word, literarily translated as *'I am what I am because of who we all are'*. Being the continent with the poorest social development indicators, pooling resources to tackle its problems is the natural way to go. But depending on poorly negotiated outside funding for its development places it in the posture of a stunted child who keeps feeding on the mother's milk even into adulthood.

This book is about the nature, trends, challenges, and perspectives of intra-state diplomacy in health in Africa. It is easy to say that the inspiration for the book has been derived from the observations of the anxiety African governments as well as the African Union Commission went through in the face of the eminently devastating coronavirus (COVID-19) that broke out in Wuhan, China, in late 2019 and had virtually brought the entire world to a standstill by mid-2020. Notwithstanding, before COVID-19, was HIV/AIDS, 65 percent of whose victims are in Africa. HIV/AIDS has ravaged the continent for over four decades now with no end in sight though AIDS-related deaths have reduced significantly because of the rampant use of cheap generic antiretroviral drugs introduced in the late 1990s. Since the epidemic started in 1981, an estimated 41 million people have died of it worldwide with 30 million in Africa. Similarly, all Ebola virus outbreaks have been in Africa where it has made most of its victims. To the surprise of all, Africa seems to have significantly minimised COVID-19 deaths, emerging as the least affected continent. This was not a coincidence when we take a look at the proactiveness of the Africa Centres for Disease Control and Prevention which had rolled out a COVID-19 pandemic protocol for testing and got the African Union to secure a provisional 270 million doses of the COVID-19 vaccine through its COVID-19 African Vaccine Acquisition Task Team (AVATT), the Africa Medical Supplies Platform (AMSP), on behalf of the Africa CDC for distribution in all AU member countries. This was the first of its kind in the history of the management of a health crisis in Africa that African and European countries secured and competed for vaccines from the same marketplaces and at the same time. This showed that the AU had positioned itself as a veritable pan-African organisation, ready to protect Africa's interests all the way. Although vaccine delivery was delayed and Africa remains the least vaccinated continent against COVID-19, the structures in the African Union notably the Africa CDC seem to be ready to respond to future disease threats to the continent if the AU's stubborn funding problems are addressed.

Like the pan-Africanists, this book posits that Africa would easily overcome most of its health problems without always first resorting to aid if the AU and member states exploit the potential for health diplomacy existing within the organisation and its regional economic communities. African Union organs like the Africa CDC, the Africa Medicine Agency, Partnerships for African Vaccines Manufacturing and many others all created since 2017 are veritable platforms for African countries to foster health cooperation and protect Africans from preventable deaths. For this to happen, African governments through the African Union Assembly and the African Union Council must commit to funding the structures they set up. This is a priority for the continent especially the countries in sub-Saharan Africa because their inability to emerge economically for over 60 years since independence can be attributed not only to the market, poor economic policies, and bad governance but also significantly to epidemics that frequently plague the continent. Whereas the economic effects of COVID-19 are still felt in many countries including even the rich ones, studies have demonstrated that epidemics like HIV/AIDS can undo many African countries' long-attained economic gains by slowing growth by up to 25 percent. The situation is even more palpable at the micro-household level where households with an HIV/AIDS patient spend twice as much on medication than other households. Children may miss school to look after sick parents thereby jeopardising their future, and less labour on the farm may result in household famine. Given the destabilising capacity of epidemics even for the rich countries, it is only through deliberate cooperation on health protection and promotion that African countries can protect their economies and their populations.

The customary pandemic response that depends on external borrowing, and the appeal for humanitarian assistance as a first step speaks poorly of a continent where crisis is not anticipated and hence not prepared for. This is a sure formula for failure.

The structure of the book includes an introduction, nine chapters, and a conclusion. The introduction seeks to situate the place of Africa in contemporary global diplomacy and to explain the historic dent in the continents' international relations with the disruptions of the Slave Trade and European imperialism which presided over the decline of many empires and kingdoms which already had long-established diplomatic practices in Africa. It explores how the continent was plagued and plundered by outside powers from the fifteenth century and only started emerging from direct colonial rule in the 1960s, consequently marking its entry into bilateral and multilateral diplomacy only 60 years ago. Finally, this section notes that the last 20 of these 60 years witnessed a remarkable shift of foreign policy objectives from strategic alliances to development in its multiple dimensions. The conclusion appraises the state of intra-African health diplomacy in general and observes the persistence of neo-colonial relations that significantly weaken the commitment of African states to continental ideals before suggesting a way forward for health diplomacy.

As health is not generally considered a core strategic objective in foreign policy, Chap. 2 examines the theoretical basis for health in foreign policy pursuits and suggests the approaches it may take. Chapter 3 gives an overview of health diplomacy in Africa from an African Union as well as the United Nations perspective. It regrets the emergence of international medical tourism to Europe, North America, and Asia practised mostly by the African elites. The author sees this as a major hindrance to the development of robust health infrastructure and the training and retaining of medical personnel on the continent—a situation inimical to intra-African health diplomacy. Chapter 4 identifies, describes, and discusses the role of regional agencies in health diplomacy on the continent. It notes the recent emergence of a plethora of health promotion and disease prevention agencies in Africa. Building on the information from Chap. 4, the fifth chapter explores the work of these agencies in implementing intra-African health diplomacy. While all chapters comment on the difficulties and challenges of implementing health diplomacy on the continent, rampant violent conflict is singled out as a major factor undermining it. That is the subject of Chap. 6 which not only discusses the causes of conflict, in general, but zooms in on the nature of the conflict in the DRC to explain how an internal conflict can generate a huge stream of refugees, jeopardise their health, yet undercut the ability of willing international partners to provide relief and healthcare. Chapter 7 examines the application of social media platforms to digital diplomacy and unveiled both the positive and negative effects on foreign policy. Drawing from the COVID-19 pandemic and others, the chapter discusses how the African Union, African leaders, and stakeholders in healthcare are using digital diplomacy in times of crisis to communicate their foreign policy. Chapter 8 raises the profile of health data sharing to highlight how international collaboration is critical in enhancing resilience to national, regional, and global public health crises. The chapter argues that having more clarity and/or understanding of the dynamics involved in international cooperation between countries or in collaborative health research is imperative for data sharing, particularly in developing economies with common health risks. The benefits of sharing health information/data which could increase healthcare delivery in Africa are outlined here. Within the framework of the global climate change debates, Chap. 9 highlights the integration of health concerns in climate change negotiations, from the African perspective. Finally, using examples mainly from the health and healthcare domain the tenth chapter attempts to argue the way forward for sub-Saharan Africa in the present global circumstances from a bioethicist viewpoint. To the author, diplomacy in this situation is likely not to be helpful because as it has been known, diplomacy appears to be an art that excels in high platitudes, equivocations, papering over nasty cracks, and valourising rather than denouncing the actual as against the possible. Hence, what must be done in and for Africa can and should be done with or without diplomacy.

London, UK   Humphrey Ngala Ndi
Coventry, UK   Henry Ngenyam Bang
London, UK   Anna Tasha Baninla Mbur
Harare, Zimbabwe   Zebulon Suifon Takwa

BOOK DESCRIPTION

The purpose of this book is to project diplomacy as an unavoidable instrument for monitoring, prevention, and control of health and disaster risks among African countries. The book advocates health cooperation in Africa at a time when pandemics are recurrent. Outside of the WHO, many countries, even within regional groupings have not actively pursued health cooperation. We intend this book to provide the basis for advocating the inclusion of health diplomacy in the curricula of the training of the African diplomat with the hope to stimulate gradual policy shifts in foreign ministries, regional groupings, and the African Union.

CONTENTS

Notes on Contributors

Henry Ngenyam Bang is a disaster risk management (DRM) scholar, educator, researcher, and practitioner. His thought leadership in DRM spans more than 15 years in the African and UK higher education systems. Currently, he teaches MSc disaster and emergency management courses at Coventry University, UK. Formerly he worked at the Bournemouth University Disaster Management Centre as a researcher and taught MSc disaster management students. Bang is an expert in African DRM and has directed research projects in West African countries while liaising with their national disaster management agencies. He has more than four dozen outputs, including academic publications in international journals, book chapters, books, and conference papers. Bang has interdisciplinary research interests including the nexus between crises and diplomacy/foreign policy. His academic profile is in Geology (BSc, MSc), and he has a second MSc (Environment and Development), and a PhD from the University of East Anglia, UK. He recently achieved a PGCE from Bournemouth University and is a Fellow of the UK Higher Education Academy.

Guy Elessa is a diplomat, serving at the High Commission for the Republic of Cameroon to the United Kingdom as First Secretary. Prior to his appointment in London, he was head of Cabinet to the Minister of External Relations (2012–2015) in Yaoundé. Education-wise, Guy Elessa holds a master's degree in public management, obtained from the University of Potsdam in German, and a master's degree in international relations, specialised in Diplomacy from the International Relations Institute of Cameroon (IRIC). He has focused his research on Africa, the

African Renaissance, and the development of African Open Strategic Autonomy. He is the author of the book *African Renaissance: South Africa's Foreign Policy and the Quest for African Development*. He has other books in preparation for publication. He is the founder of African Renaissance in the Making (ARITMA), an organisation that promotes social investment and investment in people to build a better African society.

Emmanuel Etamo Kengo is a lecturer in the Department of History and African Civilizations, University of Buea, Cameroon. He obtained his bachelor's degree in history from the University of Yaoundé. His master's degree and PhD were obtained from the Department of History and International Studies, University of Nigeria, Nsukka, in 1998 and 2007, respectively. Dr. Kengo's academic interest is in economic and social history of Africa. He has taught and supervised students in his area of interest at the University of Buea for more than a decade. He has published both internationally and locally in peer reviewed journals including chapters in edited volumes. He is a member of the African Economic History Network, and Colonial Letters Cluster of the University of Bayreuth, Germany.

Estherine Lisinge-Fotabong is the director of Programme Innovation and Planning at the African Union Development Agency (AUDA-NEPAD). In 2020, she received recognition from the Government of Egypt for her support of Africa's development and women's empowerment. In 2014 and 2016, she received honorary awards from the Governments of Ethiopia and Cameroon, respectively, for her passion, dedication, and leadership toward advancing the equality and empowerment of African women. She also received special recognition in 2015 by Top Women in Business & Government acknowledging her as a leader in agricultural policy on the continent.Before becoming director at the AUDA-NEPAD, Mrs. Fotabong was the UNEP Country Liaison Officer for South Africa and Senior Environment and Tourism Adviser to the NEPAD Secretariat. She also served as Assistant Lecturer in Law at the University of Yaoundé II, Cameroon, and as director of Policy and Strategy at WWF Central African Regional Programme Office. Mrs. Fotabong has served on several panels and international steering committees for various projects. She has co-authored several publications on climate change adaptation, and environmental law and development policy.

Humphrey Ngala Ndi is Second Counsellor (Cultural Affairs) in the High Commission for the Republic of Cameroon in London and Professor of Geography at the University of Yaoundé I, Cameroon, from where he obtained his doctorate degree in 2004. He also holds an MSc in Diplomacy and Foreign Policy from Loughborough University London. He has authored several articles in peer-reviewed journals and is a co-author of *Introduction to Health Geography* (2018). He is a member of the International Society of Global Health (ISoGH) and is affiliated to many research groups and networks. He started his career as a researcher at the National Institute of Cartography in Cameroon in 2002 before joining the University of Buea in 2008, and the University of Yaoundé I in 2013. His research interests are in the area of health geography, but he has recently developed entrenched interests in health and science diplomacy.

Zebulon Suifon Takwa currently serves as the Senior Peace and Development Advisor (PDA) with the United Nations in Zimbabwe, providing regular strategic analytical support to the Resident Coordinator and the UN Country Team in its engagement with national stakeholders in the field of peacebuilding and socio-economic development. Takwa formerly served as head of the Post-Conflict Reconstruction Unit with the African Union Commission in Addis Ababa (2009–2014). His most recent works include issue papers published by the UNDP Oslo Governance Centre, Oslo (2020), entitled: "Climate Change and Insecurity in the Lake Chad Basin: Addressing the Root Causes and Drivers of the Boko Haram Insurgency and the Herders-Farmers Conflict in Nigeria"; "Preventing Violent Conflicts in Nigeria: Challenges and Opportunities for Enhanced National Ownership" (Norwegian Institute for International Affairs—UNDP Oslo Governance Centre, Oslo, Issue paper no. 8/2017). Takwa holds a PhD, MA, and BA in History (specialisation in international relations) from the University of Yaoundé, Cameroon.

Godfrey B. Tangwa is an emeritus professor at the University of Yaoundé 1, Cameroon, where he was head of the Department of Philosophy from 2004 to 2009. He is a fellow of the Cameroon Academy of Sciences (CAS) and the African Academy of Sciences (AAS), vice chairperson of the Cameroon Bioethics Initiative (CAMBIN) which he founded in 2005, an executive committee member of the Pan-African Bioethics Initiative (PABIN), and chairperson of the Cultural, Anthropological, Social and Economic (CASE) work group of the Global Emerging Pathogens Treatment Consortium (GET). He has extensive teaching and research experience in the domains of philosophy and bioethics. He obtained a BA (1977) from the University of Nigeria, Nsukka; an MA (1979) from the University of Ife (now Obafemi Awolowo University), Ile Ife; and a PhD (1984) from the University of Ibadan, all in Nigeria. He has served on several expert advisory committees for the WHO, has been a member of the Scientific Ethics Advisory Group (SEAG) of Hoffmann La Roche since 2005, and is currently also an advisory board member of both ALERRT and SARETI. His publications' record shows about 10 books, 35 book chapters, and 45 journal articles.

Anna Baninla Mbur Tasha is currently serving as minister counsellor in the Cameroon High Commission in London, where she has equally served for some time as Charge d'affaires (February 2017 to October 2018). She is a senior diplomat, who has served for several years in the ministry of foreign affairs for the Republic of Cameroon. She is pragmatic and has acted as president of many associates for diplomatic, cultural, and social groups. As a former graduate of the International Relations Institute of Cameroon, she obtained a master's degree and a "Doctorate de troisième cycle" in International Relations. She holds a postgraduate diploma in development from the Institute of Social Studies in the Hague as well as a certificate in mediation from Align Mediation UK and is an expert in conflict prevention and management from the European Peace University Stadtschlaining, Austria. She has participated in several summits of Heads of State of the Organisation of Islamic Cooperation and of the Commonwealth Organisation.

Abbreviations and Acronyms

AEC	African Economic Community
AfCFTA	African Continental Free Trade Area
AfDB	African Development Bank
AGOA	Africa Growth and Opportunity Act
AHS	Africa Health Strategy
AID	Agency for International Development
AIDS	Acquired Immunodeficiency Syndrome
AMA	African Medicines Agency
AMCE	African Medical Centre of Excellence
AMCEN	African Ministerial Conference on Environment
AMRH	African Medicines Regulatory Harmonisation
AMU	Arab Maghreb Union
ARNS	Africa Region Nutrition Strategy
ARO	Africa Regional Office
ASI	African Solidarity Initiative
AU	African Union
AUC	African Union Commission
CAHOSSC	Committee of African Heads of State on Climate Change
CBDR-RC	Common but Differentiated Responsibilities and Respective Capacities
CC	Crisis Communication
CDC	Centre for Disease Control
CEMAC	Economic and Monetary Commission of Central African States
CFR	Case Fatality Rates
COHA	Cost of Hunger in Africa Study
COMESA	Common Market for Eastern and Southern Africa
COP	Global Climate Summit

COVAX	Covid-19 Vaccines Global Access
CVO	COVID Organics
DAC	Development Assistance Committee
DD	Digital Diplomacy
DRC	Democratic Republic of the Congo
DS	Diplomatic Signalling
EAC	East African Community
EAGLES	East African Government Leaders, Legislators, and Legal Executives
EAHRC	East African Health Research Commission
EAHSC	East African Health and Scientific Conference
ECCAS	Economic Commission of Central African States
ECHO	Extension for Community Health Outcomes
ECOWAS	Economic Community of West African States
EPG	Economic Partnership Agreements
EQUINET	Equity in Health in East and Southern Africa
ERT	Epidemic Response Team
EU	European Union
EVD	Ebola Virus Disease
FFA	Framework for Action
GCF	Green Climate Fund
GDP	Gross Domestic Product
GEF	Global Environment Facility
GHD	Global Health Diplomacy
GISAID	Global Initiative on Sharing Avian Influenza Data
GIZ	German International Cooperation Agency
HFA	Health for All
HHS	Health, Humanitarian Affairs and Social Development
HSGOC	Head of State and Government Orientation Committee
ICCO	International Cocoa Organisation
ICO	International Coffee Organisation
ICT	Information and Communication Technology
IHR	International Health Regulations
IPAA	International Partnership against AIDS in Africa
IPC	Infection Prevention and Control
IPCC	Intergovernmental Panel on Climate Change
LDC	Least Developed Countries
LIC	Low-Income Countries
LNHO	League of Nations Health Organization
MDG	Millennium Development Goals
MFA	Ministries of Foreign Affairs
MNC	Multinational Corporations

MPP	Medicines Patent Pool
NATO	North Atlantic Treaty Organisation
NCDP	National Congress for the Defence of the People
NDC	Nationally Determined Contributions
NEPAD	New Partnership for Africa's Development
NGO	Non-governmental Organisations
NHRS	National Health Research System
NIH	National Institute of Health
NWP	Nairobi Work Programme
OAU	Organisation of African Unity
OCEAC	Organization for the Coordination of the Fight Against Endemic Diseases in Central Africa
ODA	Overseas Development Assistance
OECD	Organisation for Economic Cooperation and Development
OHCA	Organization for Health in Central African Sub-region
PACT	Partnership to Accelerate COVID-19 Testing
PAVM	Partnerships for African Vaccine Manufacturing
PEPFAR	President's Emergency Plan for AIDS Relief
PHEIC	Public Health Emergency of International Concern
PMPA	Pharmaceutical Manufacturing Plan for Africa
RCC	Regional Collaborating Centres
RCUK	Research Council UK
REACH MPI	Regional East African Community Health Policy Making and Implementation
REACH RFA	Regional East African Community Health Research Funding and Accessing
RECs	Regional Economic Communities
REG	Regional Economic Groupings
RISDP	Regional Indicative Strategic Development Plan
RISLNET	Regional Integrated Surveillance and Laboratory Networks
SADC	Southern African Development Community
SAP	Structural Adjustment Programmes
SBSTA	Subsidiary Body on Scientific and Technological Advice
SSA	Sub-Saharan Africa
STC	Specialised Technical Committees
TICAD	Tokyo International Conference on African Development
TRIPS	Trade-Related Aspects of Intellectual Property Rights
UHC	Universal Health Coverage
UNAIDS	Joint United Nations Programme on HIV/AIDS
UNDP	United Nations Development Programme
UNECA	United Nations Economic Commission for Africa
UNFCCC	United Nations Framework Convention on Climate Change

UNHCR	United Nations High Commission for Refugees
UNICEF	United Nations International Children Emergency Fund
UPC	Union des Populations du Cameroun
WAHO	West African Health Organisation
WAN	Wide Area Network
WASH	Water, Sanitation and Hygiene
WHO	World Health Organisation
WOHEP	West African Health Organisation
WTO	World Trade Organisation

LIST OF FIGURES

List of Boxes

LIST OF TABLES

CHAPTER 1

Introduction

Humphrey Ngala Ndi

As a player, Africa's role in global diplomacy is virtually insignificant. This is akin to the continent's low global social, political, and economic status. According to World Bank figures from 2017, 430.83 million of the 689.11 million (62.5 percent) people living in extreme poverty in the world were in sub-Saharan Africa (SSA) (Roser & Ortiz-Ospina, 2013). Although the number of people entering extreme poverty has grown in the global south since 1990, that of Africa has been staggering. During the same period, the continent's share of global trade value (exports) stood at only 1.7 percent in 2016 (Schmieg, 2016). This is significant because, for many countries in the region, export trade accounts for more than 30 percent of gross domestic product (GDP). This proportion is even exacerbated in oil-exporting countries like Equatorial Guinea (55.1 percent), Angola (40.6 percent), Congo Brazzaville (69.1 percent), and Gabon (50.7 percent), among many others (ibid).

Despite the existence of numerous trading blocs on the continent, international trading partnerships such as the Economic Partnership

H. N. Ndi (✉)
High Commission for the Republic of Cameroon in London, London, UK

University of Yaounde I, Yaounde, Cameroon

© The Author(s), under exclusive license to Springer Nature Switzerland AG 2023
H. N. Ndi et al. (eds.), *Health Diplomacy in Africa*, Studies in Diplomacy and International Relations,
https://doi.org/10.1007/978-3-031-41249-3_1

1

Agreements (EPAs) with the European Union, the Africa Growth and Opportunity Act (AGOA) with the USA, China's numerous aid-for-trade programmes, and the Tokyo International Conference on African Development (TICAD), sub-Saharan Africa is still very marginalised in terms of global bilateral and multilateral trade. As such, it remains outside of the major networks of global capital, industry, and development (Schmieg, 2016). This is mainly due to the low value of its export trade which is dominated by primary products for which the continent receives far little money than it pays off for most of its imports constituted of processed goods.

The dismal situation of Africa's global trade value is perplexing given that the continent is home to 30 percent of the world's mineral resources (UNEP, n.d.). Africa holds 8 percent of global reserves of natural gas, 12 percent of global oil reserves, 40 percent of global gold reserves, and 90 percent of world reserves of chromium and platinum. In addition to its mineral endowments, Africa also holds over 65 percent of global arable land and 10 percent of the world's freshwater (UNEP, n.d.). As mentioned earlier, most of these resources are exported in their raw forms with very little value added to them. A case in point is the Democratic Republic of the Congo (DRC). The mineral wealth of this country provides a situation *par excellence* of a 'resource curse'. In terms of mineral wealth, it is arguably in the top 10 percent wealthiest countries in the world, but paradoxically in the bottom, 10 percent in terms of human development, ranking 174 of 189 countries (UNDP, 2020). The DRC accounts for 55 percent of the total world production of cobalt; 3.5 percent of copper; 20.5 percent of diamonds; 2.5 percent tin; 5.5 percent gemstones, and 12.4 percent tantalum (Yager, 2019).

Like in most of Africa, the mineral wealth of the DRC is exploited mainly by foreign companies which draw more benefits from the industry than the DRC. By being dominated by foreign investors, the revenue earned by these companies is mostly repatriated.

Despite its outstanding potential for economic growth and development, Africa remains an economically wobbling continent, unable to punch at its weight in global politics and diplomacy. The UNEP attempts to explain the internationally weak position of Africa by referring to the mismanagement of the continent's resources (illegal mining, logging, and fishing); illicit financial flows and capital flight; the corruption of the political and economic elites; poor political leadership; and unsound economic policies and regulations. Some of the policies that keep Africa economically backwards were initiated and continue to be sustained by African governing elites, and western multinational companies enjoying the support of their governments.

As an object or target of diplomatic manoeuvres, Africa becomes incredibly significant globally. It is courted by the richer countries with the main interest of securing adequate access to her resources, which are often carted away in poorly negotiated investment deals that do not benefit the long-term economic and social development of the continent. That explains why world economic powers justle to position themselves with Africa as the most favoured development partner through initiatives like the China-Africa, European Union-Africa, USA-Africa, and the Japan-Africa summits. Reinforcing this trend is Africa's disproportionately high burden of global disease and conflict. The frame of Africa as the land of poverty, disease, and conflict makes it the public diplomacy target of richer countries like the USA, UK, France, China, Germany, Japan, Russia, and Turkey among many others. It is not surprising, therefore, that Africa figures prominently in international development discourses, conflict prevention and management, charity outreaches, and emergency interventions from bilateral, multilateral, and non-state actors.

Africa's lopsided status in global politics has its roots in the distant historical past that has transcended all components of the continent's diplomacy and foreign policy. Taking cognisance of this diplomatic precedence for Africa, this book explores the current trends, challenges, and prospects of intra-Africa health diplomacy on the premise that robust intra-Africa relations can alter the current global system that makes Africa an object rather than a player in global affairs. In so doing, the book examines the issues that affect health cooperation among African countries and go further to discuss the prospects for health diplomacy on the continent.

A Brief Historical Review of African Diplomacy

African diplomacy predates the European colonisation of the continent. As the cradle of humanity, the natural instincts for communities to communicate, negotiate, cooperate, and engage with one another were obvious. From this perspective, Spies (2018) suggests that diplomacy was surely born in Africa. There is abundant evidence pointing to the fact that the sending of emissaries to negotiation meetings was a common practice even among people with a primitive and rudimentary culture. Examples from ancient African states like the Asante kingdom, the Ghana, Mali and

Songhai empires, and the kingdoms of Dahomey and Oyo are only a few to cite among many. These kingdoms and empires grew through conquest, trade, migration, alliances, and the integration and assimilation of others, often weaker nations, or tribal groups. Irwin (1975) notes that several states in pre-colonial Africa maintained diplomatic relations with one another in peacetime on a regular basis. Such relations were sometimes based on the rivalry as with Dahomey and Asante; on conquest as with Dahomey and Oyo; and even common ancestry and tradition as with the Yoruba and Fante states. In the early nineteenth century, the Asante king is said to have received three official embassies from the coastal kings and one each from Dahomey, Salaga, and Yendi (ibid). Within prevailing customary laws, codes of conduct evolved protocols governing the treatment of official emissaries, hosts to official guests, and the protection of strangers. It can be said that inter-state relations in Africa were governed by a system of customary international laws (Smith, 1973).

It is logical to think that the constant interactions among African states led to the emergence of a class of palace cadres knowledgeable and experienced in receiving and negotiating with foreign emissaries that they can safely be said to have been playing the role of professional diplomats. Smith (1973) equally notes that in the early European writings on West Africa, the officials of African states engaged in foreign affairs are described as ambassadors. Other words used are 'messenger'; 'linguist', and occasionally 'herald'. The coastal states entertained close relations with European settlers (traders, missionaries, and explorers). Examples abound and include the several treaties reached between Britain and the coastal kings of West Africa, notably abolishing the trade in slaves and protecting trade between them (Ardenner, 1968). Irwin (1975) points to the strong relations between the celebrated Asantehene of the Asante kingdom, in present-day Ghana with British imperialists at Cape Coast and the Dutch, at Elmina Castle. Between 1816 and 1820, the Asante king and court were visited at Kumasi, the capital of the kingdom by ten European emissaries seeking favours of one kind or the other.

Records from Cuneiform provide details of Egypt's relationships with her neighbours manifested in trading agreements, political alliances, and peaceful resolution of conflicts. The first ever written peace treaty in human history known as the Treaty of Kadesh was reached between Ramesses II, Pharoah of Egypt, and the king of the Hittites, Hattušilis III, in around 1258 BCE.

As it happened all over the world, diplomacy in pre-Westphalian Africa was often accompanied by symbolic gestures such as strategically planned marriages and high-profile visits. Marriages between princes and princesses were important in building strategic alliances and maintaining friendly relations among pre-colonial states. Kuper (1978) suggests that the female relatives of the Swazi king were considered politico-economic assets to be judiciously invested.

Although Africa was already in contact with the ancient civilizations of the Mediterranean world notably the Phoenicians, and the Middle East, before Christ, it was the European expansion into sub-Saharan Africa led by the Portuguese from the fifteenth century, generally known as the Age of Discovery, that started Europe's long-standing relationship and domination of the continent.

European expansion and imperialism that culminated in the partition of the continent in the late nineteenth century prematurely ended the splendour of African kingdoms; their statecraft and diplomatic practices as African states saw their territories carved out and coalesced with neighbouring state territories to form colonial entities under European rule and domination. The Berlin Conference of 1884–85, called to lay down the principles of the partition of Africa, sowed the seeds of the first Westphalian-styled states on the continent. After more than 80 years of colonial domination, the legal and educational systems and diplomatic practices of African kingdoms were significantly weakened and superseded by the European colonial systems. This has remained largely unchanged today even after more than 60 years of independence. After evolving into independent and self-governing territories, the African government did not decolonise the educational and legal systems, as well as their diplomatic practices the public service. Many were quick to seek diplomatic relations with their former colonial masters with a resident representative and with the more powerful countries in Europe and North America at the detriment of inter-African diplomacy. As such, the continent did not attempt to reinvent itself diplomatically, and most diplomats continued to be trained in Europe and America on a curriculum designed to serve non-African interests and to operate more like diplomatic proxies for the former colonialists.

From the creation of coastal trading posts to the exploration of the interior of the continent and eventual colonisation was not all cosy and peaceful. European colonists often used violent means to subdue African resistance and destitute their kings or chiefs to forcefully extend their rule over independent and self-governing states through the installations of more moderate puppet rulers. Where some African rulers could not stand up to the superior firearms of the Europeans, they agreed to treaties extending European rule and protection over their populations and territories. The decline of pre-colonial political, economic, and military power meant that African diplomacy gradually passed into the hands of the colonists who had rendered the kings and chiefs subservient to them.

With the colonisation of Africa nearly complete by 1914, African diplomacy naturally passed into the hands of the imperialists. The imperial powers created new states generally bigger in territory and population than the pre-colonial states. In this new dispensation, the diplomatic powers of the African kings and chiefs became inconsequential. The colonies with new and arbitrary boundaries were administered as outposts of the imperial governments in Europe and this period overwhelmingly wreaked havoc on Africa's socio-political systems as it rolled back the diplomatic prowess African kings, queens, and chiefs had achieved from centuries of interacting as sovereigns with other states, Arabs, Europeans, Chinese, and Indians.

The Portuguese set out with the objective of finding a sea route to India but also established coastal trading posts on the continent as they came into contact with it. Among the earliest of such posts were Al Mina (the mine) also called Elmina today (1469), Fernâo do Pó (1472) (Fernando Po) today called Bioko, São Tome (1485), Diogo Câo (1482), Zanzibar (1583), and the kingdom of Nwenemutapa in the sixteenth century. Trade with Africans was usually preceded by negotiations and treaties reached with native leaders (kings, chiefs) who exercised real territorial sovereignty over their kingdoms or states and who controlled trade with the hinterlands. The peace treaty negotiated with Queen Nzinga of the Ambundu kingdoms of Ndongo and Matamba, located in present-day northern Angola; the kingdom of Nwenemutapa, as well as the Zanzibari and Swahili chiefs of east Africa are just a few examples of the diplomatic relations pre-colonial African states entertained with early Europeans on the continent. Much has been written on the diplomatic prowess of African kings and queens in general and the resistance staged by Queen Nzinga (Nzinga Mbande) against the Portuguese who sought to expand slave trading into Central Africa (Bortolot, 2003).

AFRICA IN COLONIAL TO POST-COLONIAL DIPLOMACY

Diplomacy in the post-Westphalian era has been defined as the application of intelligence and tact to the conduct of official relations between the governments of sovereign states through peaceful means. Inherent in the concept of peace is the ability to negotiate or deal with differences without resorting to force. Although diplomacy is predicated on the peaceful conduct of relations among states, guided by tact, intelligence and wisdom, how successful negotiations are depend on the ability of states to apply subtle pressures on each other, all backed up, of course by the level of real economic, military, or cultural power behind them. Whereas negotiations are a key element in diplomatic practice, the influence of Niccolò Machiavelli, an Italian author, diplomat, philosopher, and historian, introduced the use of a complex range of clever ruses, moral, deceitful, and psychological weapons in negotiations in a conflict situation (Booth-Gore & Pakenham, 1979).

For the 75 years of her subjugation (1885 to 1960), for most colonial territories, Africa's most visible phases internationally were the First and the Second World Wars fought between 1914–1918 and 1939–1945, respectively. Crowder (1985) notes that a million African soldiers were involved in the wars in Europe. Men and women were often forcibly recruited as carriers to support the supply lines of European armies fighting on the continent, in Europe, and elsewhere. Africa lost an estimated 150,000 soldiers and carriers in the First World War. African soldiers were also used by the colonists in quelling rebellions that had erupted in many territories, weakened by the World Wars. There were revolts in Libya, Southern Ivory coast, Karamoja in Uganda, and Dahomeyan Borgu, among others. When World War I ended, all African soldiers involved were committed to one side or the other, but predominantly to the Allied or Entente powers led by France, the United Kingdom, Russia, Italy, Japan, and the United States, against the Central Powers led by Germany, Austria-Hungary, the Ottoman Empire, and Bulgaria. The Versailles Peace Treaty that ended the war had consequences that still reverberate in some former German colonies in Africa notably Cameroon and Togoland. A similar scenario occurred in the Second World War where the British conscripted and deployed over 80 000 British West African soldiers in Burma, while the French enlisted over 100 000 African soldiers in Europe and other parts of their colonial empire.

During these wars African soldiers were the most visible expression of the continent's contribution to the existing international order. Perhaps, the greatest benefit of the Second World War to Africa was the economic and military decline of France and Britain, the greatest empire builders on the continent. Byfield et al. (2015) reveal that Africans exploited these weaknesses and increasingly demanded their rights in deciding their futures, their rights as workers, and an end to the indignities of racism. The reliance on Africans to fight on their sides also revealed a weakness in the colonists that had not been known to the Africans before. The involvement of the United States of America, and her stance against colonial subjugation, is reflected in the Atlantic Charter agreed upon between President Franklin Roosevelt and British Prime Minister Winston Churchill, in 1941, setting the stage for British decolonisation. In its third article, the signatories to the Charter agreed to '...respect the right of all peoples to choose the form of government under which they will live; and … to see sovereign rights and self-government restored to those who have been forcibly deprived of them'.

Between 1941 and 1968, Britain and France, who had the greatest number of colonial possessions in Africa, granted independence to over 33 territories between them with 29 in the 1960s, explaining why that period is often described as the independence decade. This period marked a new beginning for African diplomacy. The early 1960s were crucial times for Africa and the United Nations because 21 newly independent African territories (now sovereign countries) were admitted into the United Nations Organisation (UNO) between 1960 and 1962 marking Africa's debut in multilateral diplomacy. The need for concerted effort in international affairs was immediately felt by the newly independent African countries, especially with the advocacy of pan-Africanist leaders like Dr Kwame Nkrumah of Ghana and Emperor Haile Selassie of Ethiopia.

The processes of a viable state and empire formation having been nipped in the bud by colonisation, few independent African countries were nation-states. Eventually, independence was granted to countries whose boundaries were arbitrarily drawn at Berlin in 1884–85 carving out territories harbouring small-sized precolonial African kingdoms, or empires. The immediate implication of this feature of African countries was the dearth of a national feeling as ethnicity and tribalism remained strong, rendering the states weak. Fully aware of this scenario, the need for Africa to speak with one strong voice in the world was echoed in the creation of the Organisation of African Unity (OAU) on 25 May 1963 in

Addis Ababa with thirty-two signatories, twenty-two of which had acceded to independence between 1960 and 1963. In the same light, 21 African countries were admitted into the United Nations Organisation between 1960 and 1962. The most significant reform of the UN Security Council is said to have been orchestrated by the huge number of African countries joining the organisation in the 1960s. Like Spies (2018) puts it, the sheer magnitude of decolonisation in the second part of the twentieth century driven mostly by the birth of dozens of African countries triggered the only ever reform of the UN Security Council which entailed an enlargement of the number of elected and non-permanent members of the organ from six to ten. The OAU did not attempt to revisit colonial African boundaries drawn up in Europe with disregard for the prevailing ethnic, political, and natural realities on the ground. The inheritance and ratification of colonial boundaries by the OAU played to the neo-colonial interests of the colonists.

There is no doubt that at independence, African states in general had great diplomatic ambitions. This is evident from the speed at which they adhered to the OAU now the African Union (AU) and the UNO. At Ghana's independence, Kwame Nkrumah declared inter alia 'we are going to demonstrate to the world, to the other nations, that we are prepared to lay our foundation—our own African personality'. The forebears of the AU were not only interested in liberating the continent from colonial domination when the OAU Charter was adopted in 1963 but to forge a new image and place for the continent in the world. Article two of the OAU Charter states the resolve of African countries to coordinate and harmonise their policies in many domains including cooperation in health, sanitation, and nutrition and specialised commissions composed of relevant ministers from member states were charged with the duty of implementing these resolutions. The Lagos Plan of Action for the economic development of Africa, among many points, also underscored the need for African countries to seek indigenous solutions to their health woes. It encouraged African countries to seek holistic health care for the continent's communities particularly the poorest within the context of integrated rural development. It also encouraged the development of environmentally and culturally sound technologies, to ensure that essential drugs are manufactured at low costs and from indigenous materials, and health information is regularly exchanged with other countries (OAU, 1980).

Despite the diplomatic ambitions of early African leaders, a multitude of factors militated against their ability to influence the course of international politics in their favour. The dearth of diplomatic training and skilled diplomats rendered them inept to articulate and cogently pursue the interests of their countries in international organisations and host countries. The few countries with training institutions for diplomats emphasized strategic international power politics and diplomatic protocol in their curricula at the expense of relevant domains like international economics and finance. This scenario was further weakened by a gaunt government bureaucracy, manned by civil servants performing mainly clerical duties, while the responsibility to conceive and restructure the civil service remained solidly in the hands of the international civil servants working in government ministries within different cooperation frameworks usually with the former colonist, pushing their own subtle interests. With the precedence described above, post-colonial diplomatic practices in many African countries remained colonial as they were thought out and implemented by the *cooperants* in francophone Africa, and *expats* in Anglophone Africa and implemented by an emerging elites educated mainly in European universities. Although framed in attractive international development terms that denoted the desire to help the newly independent countries, the avowed long-term strategic goals of western scholarship were mostly perverse and aimed at training like-minded elites who will be sympathetic to the public diplomacy interests of the colonist. Thus flourished many scholarship schemes administered by the *Cooperation Française* and the British Council, just to mention only these two. African countries were unable to indigenise education and administration in part because of the colonial educational systems they continued to pursue. Strongly linked to this was the inability to use African languages in schools and the civil service. Rather, more credit and praise were accorded to those educated in western universities while those educated at home were despised. To date, Africans still strongly identify as Anglophone, Francophone, Lusophone, and Hispanic.

Neo-colonial ties have continued to evolve in character and content and remain a major hindrance to the continent's ability to brand itself diplomatically. French economic recovery after the Second World War drew enormously from her African colonies and General Charles de Gaulle genuinely believed that the colonial empire would remain French, with the total exclusion of the idea of autonomy and evolution outside the French bloc (Smith & Jeppesen, 2017). To the colonist, independence for

Africa simply meant adjustment and compromises by the European colonial masters and settler populations to contain claims of 'African nationalism' (Hodgkin, 1956, cited in Smith & Jeppesen, 2017). This colonial mindset has been subtly and intricately developed and characterise relationships between France and its former African colonies and has evolved into what is usually described as *France-Afrique*.

Resident diplomatic missions are an expensive endeavour, and few African countries have a global diplomatic reach. As such, many countries on the continent prefer multilateral diplomacy through continental, regional, as well as international organisations where they are called upon to contribute membership dues in order to participate substantively. As many countries struggle to pay, they find their representatives voiceless and unable to participate in reaching major decisions. In addition, because richer European, North American, and Asian countries contribute more to these organisations, a patron-client relationship often emerges where the weaker members find themselves dictated to in the organisations. This patron-client relationship transcends nearly all of Africa's diplomatic relationships with former colonists. The case of the international governance of Africa's commodities is palpable. Even though coffee and cocoa are produced in the tropics where most developing countries are located, the International Coffee Organization (ICO) is headquartered in London, and the International Cocoa Organisation (ICCO) was only recently relocated to Abidjan in Cote d'Ivoire in 2017, after being headquartered for 44 years in London.

No sooner was Africa liberated from colonial domination than the manifestations of the Cold War engulf the continent. Tensions between communist and democratic forms of government strained relations between the USA and the USSR providing the ideological underpinnings of the Cold War. The developing countries (mostly former colonies) in Africa, Asia, and South America became critical for both powers to expand their spheres of influence. Fearing that newly independent African countries may come under communist or capitalist influences, many proxy conflicts between the former USSR and the USA and their allies erupted on the continent. The most illustrated of these conflicts was in the Belgian Congo (now the Democratic Republic of the Congo) where Patrice Emery Lumumba, the first Prime Minister was forced out of office and assassinated by US and Belgian security operatives for his nationalist stands for accepting military assistance from the USSR. He was replaced by a pro-Western leader. Other significant Cold War proxy conflicts included the Angolan Civil War (1975 to 2002) and several military takeovers. These instabilities significantly destabilised and blighted Africa's global reputation as a viable diplomatic partner. That perception of the continent remains strong among Western diplomats and politicians today especially as there has been a recrudescence of military coups on the continent in the past five years.

Africa's ability to entertain equal and strong diplomatic relations was further wrecked by persistent international indebtedness. The commodity boom in the immediate post-independence period had given African leaders the leverage to engage ambitious public sector spending on infrastructure, import substitution industries, and social projects. That did not last long because commodity prices started plummeting in the early 1970s. The direct consequence was a fall in foreign exchange earnings and a deteriorating balance of trade and payment. The lack of liquidity to run public services pushed many African countries to seek loans often on high-interest rates from international finance institutions and richer nations, especially with the expansion of the Eurodollars. This was compounded by the oil shocks of 1973–1974 and the inflationary pressures it brought to bear on young African countries and governments. The entry of Africa into international indebtedness significantly diminished its economic and political sovereignty as some economies had to be financed almost entirely through borrowing, accompanied by strong conditions that gave the lender preference in trade and investment. Thus, rather than indigenising their businesses, economies in the former African colonies rapidly passed into foreign hands when multilateral donors imposed economic liberalisation as a key condition for structural adjustment borrowing.

Added to this, is the lack of monetary independence for the former French colonies in Africa who still use the Franc CFA currency which was pegged initially to the French Franc and now the Euro at a fixed parity guaranteed by compulsory deposits by these countries of 50 percent of their foreign exchange earnings in the French treasury. In this way, these countries are economically subservient to the French who control their monetary policy as well as their ability to freely diversify their international partners. Although some economists and politicians argue that the arrangement guarantees a stable currency for these African countries, the negative effects on the international competitivity of these economies are far reaching because of fix-parity high-valued currency not backed by production. These countries cannot freely devalue their currencies to render their exports competitive and cannot easily engage import substitution policies. Briefly, their economic and political sovereignties decline as do their international diplomatic leverages.

As outlined in the preceding paragraphs, Africa's post-colonial diplomatic visibility was compromised by superpower Cold War rivalries on the continent, the debt crisis, and the inability of an ill-adapted OAU to convey and implement the continent's economic and political vision. The Lagos Plan Action for the development of Africa formulated in 1980 is considered the first effort to push the OAU's agenda beyond liberating the continent from the vestiges of colonialisation as articulated at creation in 1963. Regretting the dismal economic growth record of the continent in the twenty years following independence, the Plan can be said to be the first comprehensive blueprint for the development of the continent. Among other things, it determined to undertake measures for the basic restructuring of the economic base of the continent and to adopt a far-reaching regional approach based primarily on collective self-reliance. Africa's regional groupings are practical laboratories for intra-African diplomacy, which is still, nevertheless, held back from blossoming because of overlapping memberships, the lack of will to contribute financially to the organisations, and continued strong undermining economic ties by some countries to their former colonial masters. This is evident in the Francophone spheres—Economic Commission of Central African States (ECCAS) and Monitory Commission of Central African States (CEMAC), where integration illustrated by the free movement of goods, services, and people still lags far behind the other regional groupings on the continent.

The end of minority rule in Zimbabwe in 1980, the end of the Cold War and dissolution of the Soviet Union in December 1991, and the release of the anti-apartheid icon, Nelson Mandela from prison culminated at the end of white minority rule in South Africa in 1994, marked a new era for the OAU as it had exhausted it political liberation agenda (Spies, 2018). The organisation had to define new objectives for the continent facing up to its dismal governance records, fostering peace and security, and promoting social and economic development. These vision goals could not be achieved within the framework of the 1963 OAU Charter. Under the impetus of charismatic leaders like Nigeria's Olusegun Obasanjo and South Africa's Thabo Mbeki, a new organisation was conceived to succeed the OAU. In 2000, the Constitutive Act creating the African Union was adopted.

In a bid to render the AU more proactive in African development, the New Economic Partnership for Africa's Development (NEPAD) was adopted at the 37th session of the Assembly of Heads of State and Governments in July 2001 in Lusaka, Zambia. It was subsequently integrated into AU structures with the vision to build an integrated, prosperous and peaceful Africa driven from within by its own citizens to represent a dynamic force in the global arena. It also has the mission to work with African countries, both individually and collectively towards sustainable growth and development. NEPAD became the AU's socio-economic flagship programme, with the quadruple objectives of eradicating poverty, promoting sustainable growth and development, integrating Africa into the global economy, and empowering African women. The structure has a Head of State and Government Orientation Committee (HSGOC) composed of 20 members including the five founding members of NEPAD—South Africa, Nigeria, Algeria, Egypt, and Senegal. The fifteen remaining members are elected to the HSGOC on a two-year rotative basis following the five AU regional groupings. Among the numerous initiatives of NEPAD is the African Medicines Regulatory Harmonisation (AMRH) programme which aims to improve access to high quality and safe drugs for African citizens by promoting the harmonisation of medicines regulations among African countries through RECs. In July 2018, at the 31st Ordinary Session of the Assembly of African Union Heads of State and Government in Nouakchott, Mauritania, a decision was taken to transform the NEPAD Agency into the first development agency of the African Union—AUDA-NEPAD, with a strengthened mandate to fast-track the realisation of Agenda 2063.

Africa, the African Union, and Health Diplomacy

While archaeological evidence points to the occurrence of epidemics in pre-colonial Africa (Chirikure, 2020; Ogundiran, 2020), little is known about how different kingdoms, empires or city-states cooperated among themselves to control or manage them. There is also archaeological evidence to show that at this time in Africa, different strategies for dealing with epidemics or pandemics existed (Chirikure, 2020).

Notwithstanding, as indicated earlier, geopolitical changes in the last quarter of the twentieth century marked by the demise of the USSR and the emergence of a unipolar world released resources hitherto trapped in financing geostrategic activities to a renewed interest in democracy, governance, and development. In 1986, through a General Assembly resolution (41/128), the United Nations embraced the fact that development was an inalienable universal human right in which all people were entitled to participate and to enjoy (United Nations General Assembly (UNGA), 1986). Taking the queue from the Lagos Plan of Action (1980) for the development of Africa to the Abuja Treaty of 1991 establishing the African Economic Community (AEC), the African Union (AU) constitutive act was agreed on 11 July 2000 in Lomé, Togo to replace the Organisation of African Unity which had existed since 1963. Among the many objectives of the AU was the resolve to cooperate with international partners to eradicate preventable diseases and promote good health on the continent. With this orientation, the AU has been able to achieve significant milestones in the prevention and treatment of diseases like HIV/AIDS, the Ebola virus disease (EVD) and others. The organisation has built up a strong network of institutions working for health prevention and protection on the continent. These include the Africa Centre for Disease Control and Prevention, a specialised technical institution of the AU established to support public health initiatives of member states and strengthen the capacity of their public health institutions to detect, prevent, control, and respond quickly and effectively to disease threats. The African Medicines Agency (AMA) is the most recent addition to the continent's health diplomacy institutions. It was established in 2019 by the Africa Union Assembly to succeed the African Medicines Regulatory Harmonisation Initiative (AMRH). It is a move to harmonise medicine regulatory framework at the continental level. In 2020, the treaty setting up AMA was ratified by 15 African countries. Health diplomacy as soft power can offer strong strategic influence and advantage in international relations. A case in point is the US President's Emergency Strategic Plan for AIDS Relief (PEPFAR) approved in 2003. With nearly US$ 65 billion PEPFAR is the biggest single-disease global initiative in history (Daschle & Frist, 2015). Healthy populations provide more productive labour and stable societies. Paraphrasing President Obama's National Security Strategy, the United States is safer and stronger when fewer people face destitution, when our trading partners are flourishing, and when societies are freer. Good health is the running thread through economic, political, and social prosperity. A poor population is a recipe for instability, refugee movements, and the destabilisation of society. It is overtly true, therefore, that health diplomacy is not an outlier in today's foreign policy objectives of any country that is desirous of safeguarding its security and stability.

Whereas the benefits of stronger cooperation in health are very apparent to individual African countries as well as the African Union, major obstacles to the full blossom of health diplomacy on the continent remain strong. They derive principally from the dearth of political will by AU member states to commit fully to the ideals of the organisation as a veritable pan-African structure. As long as the AU cannot be auto-financed through memberships dues; depend on financing from foreign entities which have their own strategic foreign policy interests in Africa; and continue to prioritise neo-colonial relationships like the Commonwealth of Nations and the Francophonie over pan-African interest, her diplomatic prowess will remain in the doldrums of global politics.

REFERENCES

African Union. (2000, July 11). Constitutive Act of the African Union. African Union. https://au.int/sites/default/files/pages/34873-file-constitutiveact_en.pdf

Ardenner, S. G. (1968). *Eyewitnesses to the annexation of Cameroon 1883–1887* (1st ed.). Ministry of Primary Education and West Cameroon Antiquities Commission.

Booth-Gore, L., & Pakenham, D. (1979). *Satow's guide to diplomatic practice*. Longman.

Bortolot, A. I. (2003). Women leaders in African history: Ana Nzinga, Queen of Ndongo. https://www.scott.k12.ky.us/userfiles/2458/Classes/15149/ana%20nzinga,%20pedro%20naranjo,%20maroons.pdf?id=78794

Byfield, J., Brown, C. A., Rarsons, T., & Sikainga, A. A. (2015). *Africa and World War II*. Cambridge University Press. https://doi.org/10.1017/CBO9781107282018

Chirikure, S. (2020, May 4). Archeology shows how ancient African societies managed pandemics. *The Conversation*. https://theconversation.com/archaeology-shows-how-ancient-african-societies-managed-pandemics-138217#:~:text=Analysis%20of%20archaeological%20evidence%20reveals,shifting%20homesteads%20to%20new%20locations

Crowder, M. (1985). The first world war and its consequences. In A. Boahen (Ed.), *General history of Africa, Vol. VII. Africa under colonial domination 1880–1935* (pp. 307–335). UNESCO.

Daschle, T., & Frist, B. (2015). The case for the strategic health diplomacy: A study of PEPFAR. Bipartisan Policy Center. https://bipartisanpolicy.org/download/?file=/wp-content/uploads/2019/03/BPC_Strategic-Health-November-2015.pdf

Hodgkin, T. (1956). Nationalism in colonial Africa. *Sudan Notes and Records, 37*(1956), 126–130. http://www.jstor.org/stable/41716729

Irwin, G. W. (1975). Pre-colonial African diplomacy: The example of Asante. *The International Journal of African Historical Studies, 8*(1), 81–96.

Kuper, A. (1978). Rank and preferential marriage in Southern Africa: The Swazi. *Man, 13*(4), 567–579. https://doi.org/10.2307/2801249

OAU. (1963, May 25). OAU Charter. The Organisation of African Unity. https://au.int/sites/default/files/treaties/7759-file-oau_charter_1963.pdf

OAU. (1980). Lagos plan of action for the Economic Development of Africa 1980–2000. Organisation of African Unity. https://www.merit.unu.edu/wp-content/uploads/2015/01/Lagos-Plan-of-Action.pdf

Ogundiran, A. (2020). Managing epidemics in ancestral Yoruba towns and cities: "Sacred groves" as isolation sites. *African Archaeological Review, 37*(3), 497–502. https://doi.org/10.1007/s10437-020-09407-5

Roser, M., & Ortiz-Ospina, E. (2013). Global extreme poverty. https://ourworldindata.org/poverty

Schmieg, E. (2016). Africa's position in global trade—Free trade agreements, WTO and regional integration. https://www.swp-berlin.org/publications/products/projekt_papiere/Africas_Position_in_Global_Trade.pdf

Smith R. (1973). Peace and palaver: international relations in pre-colonial west africa. *Journal of African History, 14*(4), 599–621.

Smith, A. W., & Jeppesen, C. (2017). *Britain, France and the decolonisation of Africa: Future imperfect?* UCL Press. https://doi.org/10.2307/j.ctt1mtz521

Spies, Y. K. (2018). African diplomacy. In G. Martel (Ed.), *The Encyclopaedia of diplomacy.* https://doi.org/10.1002/9781118885154.dipl0005

UNDP. (2020). Human Development Report 2020: The next frontier. https://hdr.undp.org/content/human-development-report-2020

UNEP. (n.d.). Our work in Africa. https://www.unep.org/regions/africa/our-work-africa#:~:text=Africa%20is%20home%20to%20some,of%20its%20chromium%20and%20platinum

UNGA. (1986). Declaration on the Right to Development. Resolution 41/128, 97th plenary meeting. https://www.ohchr.org/Documents/Issues/Development/DeclarationRightDevelopment_en.pdf

Yager, T. R. (2019). The Mineral Industry of Congo (Kinshasa): 2015 Mineral Yearbook, USGS. https://d9-wret.s3.us-west-2.amazonaws.com/assets/palladium/production/atoms/files/myb3-2015-congo-kinshasha.pdf

CHAPTER 2

Health in Diplomacy and Foreign Policy

Humphrey Ngala Ndi

INTRODUCTION

Traditionally, diplomacy is perceived and practised within the framework of power relations among sovereign states. Viewed as such by ministries of foreign affairs, concerns relating to social development are often farfetched from the traditional diplomat. That may explain why health as a 'stand-alone' subject has tended to be peripheric in diplomatic discourse and is likely to be important only in the dimension in which it may affect states' political and economic security (Loewenson et al., 2014). Thus, conceptualising the integration of health as a key component of conventional diplomacy seems illusionary to the theoretical diplomat. In the past two decades, classical diplomacy's context, content, practices, and procedures have evolved tremendously under the irresistible influence of internet technology and its spinoffs of instantaneous virtual communication at the reach of multiple stakeholders, most of whom have no formal training or experience in diplomatic protocol. This current has been styled 'track two diplomacy' where the non-state actors notably non-governmental

H. N. Ndi (✉)
High Commission for the Republic of Cameroon in London, London, UK

University of Yaounde I, Yaounde, Cameroon

H. N. Ndi et al. (eds.), *Health Diplomacy in Africa*, Studies in Diplomacy and International Relations,
https://doi.org/10.1007/978-3-031-41249-3_2

organisations and charities, diaspora organisations, and individuals engage each other internationally over subjects ranging from human rights, health and social development, investments, agriculture, to climate change. The democratisation of diplomatic space especially with the advent of track two diplomacy and the recognition of the health risk of fast global travel and trade have enhanced interests in global and international health.

Health diplomacy has become important in foreign policy discourse basically because of the renewed importance of *global health* and *international health* in the post-Cold War era. The proof of its increasing effervescence is seen in the number and diversity of publications (books, journal articles) in global health in international relations in the past few years (Davies et al., 2014). In order to avoid any confusion in the use of the terms global health and international health, it is important to elucidate the basic distinctions that have emerged between the two concepts. Global health is defined by Koplan et al. (2009), as an area of study, research, and practice that prioritises the improvement of health and the attainment of health equity for all people worldwide. This is reasonably similar to the view of global health as addressing issues and engaging practices that transcend national boundaries with a focus on global forces that determine the health of all people (Kickbush, 2006); worldwide enhancement of health; levelling up of health disparities; and protection against global threats that disregard national borders (Macfarlane et al., 2008). International health on its part has been referred to as the application of public health principles to the problems and challenges that affect low- and middle-income countries usually in the forms of development aid and humanitarian assistance. Koplan et al. (2009) have anchored these distinctions based on geographical coverage, level of international cooperation, individuals or communities, access to health, and range of disciplines involved as illustrated in Table 2.1.

A detailed review of global health and international health is important because they are implicitly facilitated and implemented by diplomats in bilateral or multilateral settings. As such, health diplomats work for global health, through global organisations like the World Health Organization (WHO), or international health as in the case of international development agencies, non-governmental organisations, and multiple bilateral and multilateral arrangements.

Another observation has been that most global health and international agencies are often based in the richer economies and the health solutions they seek for populations or individuals mainly target the poorer countries.

Table 2.1   The comparison of global, international, and public health

	Global Health	International Health	Public Health
Geographical coverage	Focuses on issues that directly or indirectly affect health but that can transcend national boundaries	Focuses on health issues of countries other than one's own, especially those of low-income and middle-income	Focuses on issues that affect the health of the population of a particular community or country
Level of cooperation	Conception, elaboration, and implementation of health solutions often require global cooperation	Conception, elaboration, and implementation of solutions usually require bilateral cooperation	Conception, elaboration, and implementation of solutions do not usually require international cooperation
Individuals or communities	Takes on both prevention in populations and clinical care of individuals	Takes on both prevention in populations and clinical care of individuals	Mainly focuses on prevention programmes for populations
Access to health	Health equity among nations and for all people is a prime objective	Seeks to enhance the health of people, especially in low-income countries	Health equity within the country or community is a key consideration
Interdisciplinarity	Highly interdisciplinary and multidisciplinary within and beyond health sciences	Embraces a few disciplines but does not emphasise multidisciplinary	Encourages multidisciplinary approaches within health sciences and with the social sciences

Source: Koplan et al. (2009)

As important as health may be in international cooperation, makers of health policies, often bureaucrats in ministries of public health and allied practitioners notably researchers and charities, have failed to understand that the principles and calculations in foreign policy are framed around issues of national interest that dominantly centre on the need for sovereign states to survive and grow in an anarchical international space where the lack of a generally accepted superpower or leviathan responsible for maintaining order means that countries are responsible for the protection of their sovereignties (Fidler, 2009). Because states are always competing with each other to safeguard their national interests, matters of sovereignty and security, often supersede social concerns like health and education. Consequently, it would seem health in the context of international cooperation is better accommodated within international development, international health, or global health. The frontiers of health in foreign policy may not expand greatly in an international system where the need for peace and security supersedes every other concern. Diplomats are more preoccupied with threats of a nuclear meltdown in the event of a major war, international terrorism, the refugee and migration crisis, all events that can undermine state sovereignty and security, than health, although the increasing frequency of deadly pandemics is also fast becoming a formidable threat to state security and survival.

Despite these realist considerations, the neoliberal ideology and the emergence of global health and international health have given a lease of life as well as sustained the important status many states now accord to issues of health especially the prevention and control of infectious diseases. Statements of intent like the 2007 Oslo Ministerial Declaration on global health have also provided a strong basis to advocate for health in diplomacy and foreign policy. To model health as an important foreign policy objective, Fidler (2005), Kickbusch et al. (2021), Kickbusch (2013); Kickbusch et al. (2013), Labonté (2014), Smith et al. (2010), Felbaum et al. (2010), Felbaum and Michaud (2010) have developed frameworks within which health can be analysed as a strategic interest in foreign policy.

The Framework for Health in Foreign Policy

Fidler (2005) has conceptualised three ways by which health can be considered in foreign policy analysis: regression, remediation, or revolution.

As a *regression*, health is considered a security issue and prevails over public health rules and principles. In this case, an epidemic is seen as a possible disruptive force to regional or cross-border economic activity and not just in its own right as a problem that impairs the quality of life of a people. The reasoning here is that limiting movements and economic activity to curb a pandemic, for example, may result in economic recession producing undesirable effects like social strife and unrest that undermines public security with the potential to bring down a government and destabilise a whole country or region. In the 2020–2021 COVID-19 response around the world, there have been numerous protests staged against lockdowns across Europe and North America. An anti-COVID-19 protest across major cities in China in November 2022 was not perceived as a light threat to president Zi Jinping's government, forcing it to lessen the stringency of the lockdown measures which had been instituted since the start of the pandemic.

As *remediation*, health issues are addressed through the conduits or hierarchies of conventional diplomacy and foreign policy but with no special role in international relations. In recognition of the importance and technical complexity of global health negotiations, some countries have created a diplomatic position for a health *attaché* in the organisational chart of their diplomatic missions. Others have seconded diplomats to international health departments like the WHO and UNICEF (Kickbusch et al., 2007). The regional groupings in Africa all have specialised agencies for health protection and promotion—the West African Health Organisation (WOHEP) in ECOWAS and the East African Community Health Department, among others.

In *revolution*, health is positioned as a right, goal, and shared global responsibility with a profound transformative role in diplomacy and foreign policy. The revolutionary perspective positions health as a global human right. This aligns with the position the UN took on addressing the extent of the HIV/AIDS pandemic worldwide and particularly in Africa in Security Council Resolution 1308 of 17 July 2000 (United Nations Security Council, 2000).

Diplomacy is a dynamic profession whose practitioners must move along with the challenges of the time. It finds itself at the essence of global as well as international health. As such, modern diplomats do not only engage their host governments and partners with matters of power politics but also negotiate issues related to social justice and transborder security, a lot of which revolves around health. Kickbusch (2011) following Fidler (2005) has identified four ways in which foreign policy and health can interact:

1. Foreign policy can endanger health when diplomacy breaks down or when trade considerations negate health outcomes. When two countries indulge in cross-border hostilities, joint immunisation campaigns suffer resulting in the endemicity of diseases like polio, yellow fever, and many others.
2. Health can be used as an instrument of foreign policy to achieve other goals such as trading health assistance for better economic cooperation in resource-rich countries of Africa.

3. Health is considered an integral part of foreign policy. In her tenure as US Secretary of State, Hillary Clinton created the Office of Global Health Diplomacy (OGHD) to advance US policy on global health.
4. Foreign policy may be used to promote health goals, where social development is a central component of a country's diplomacy.

Health in diplomacy has been described as the radar of foreign policy and positioned centrally to three global agendas:

- Security, driven by the fear of global pandemics and biological warfare where pathogens are spread intentionally.
- The effects of poor health on development; pandemics on global markets but also the widening gains accruing to pharmaceutical companies in drugs such as the antiretrovirals, and antimalarials.
- Using foreign policy to reinforce health as social justice and a human right via the support for UN initiatives like the Millennium Development Goals and the Sustainable Development Goals.

For Labonté (2014) six compelling reasons justify the importance of health in foreign policy practice. Health is seen as security (national, economic, and human); health as a major preoccupation in international development; health as a global public good; health as trade; health as a human right; and health as an ethical or moral imperative.

To crown it, the UN Secretary-General defined the basic functions of foreign policy in the twenty-first century as 'achieving security, creating economic wealth, supporting development in low-income countries and protecting human dignity' (UNGA, 2009). Whereas this subscribes to the tradition of international health, there seems to be no better way of protecting human dignity than by protecting human health, which itself is an essential economic resource.

The views of Fidler (2005), Kickbusch (2011), Labonté (2014) and Labonté and Gagnon (2010) might have been influenced by liberal internationalist thought which gained traction after the end of the Cold War when the bipolar geostrategic rivalry between the USA and the USSR came to an end, as the latter ceased to exist. Liberal internationalists believe that international progress among peoples and countries is possible, where *progress* is defined as a movement toward increasing levels of harmonious political, economic, and social cooperation among countries. This is akin to soft power diplomacy advocated by Nye (2004), where the promotion of common interests and values to attract and persuade should take prominence over the use of hard military power to coerce and influence other nations. However, the absence of international conflict does not automatically translate into international peace, harmony, and progress because political conditions in individual sovereign states may profoundly affect the ability of these countries to meet the basic social needs of their populations.

Though these frameworks strongly advocate the case for and benefits of health in foreign policy considerations, it is the framework for science diplomacy developed by the American Association for the Advancement of Science (AAAS) in conjunction with the Royal Society that provides a context within which the frontiers of the subject can be explored systematically. Dr Nina Federoff, Science and Technology Adviser to the US Secretary of State, defines science diplomacy as the use of scientific interactions among nations to address the common problems facing humanity and to build constructive, knowledge-based international partnerships (Royal Society, 2010). As the Rt Hon Gordon Brown, former Prime of the UK observed, 'many of the challenges we face today are international and—whether it's tackling climate change or fighting disease—these global problems require global solutions' (ibid.).

The report of a meeting on 'New frontiers in science diplomacy' hosted by the Royal Society in 2009 in partnership with the AAAS and attended by about 200 delegates (government ministers, scientists, diplomats, policymakers, business leaders, and journalists) from Africa, Asia, and North and South America suggested three paradigmatic dimensions of science diplomacy, which can be adapted for health diplomacy analysis too. These are science in diplomacy, diplomacy for science, and science for diplomacy.

Science in diplomacy should ensure the effective uptake of advice by policymakers. The scientific community in its diversity must inform the policymakers with up-to-date information on the dynamics of the earth's natural and socio-economic systems including health. They must also identify areas where knowledge is inadequate or uncertain (Royal Society, 2010). In the specific case of *health in diplomacy*, this approach suggests that health can be an important component in the pursuit of a country's strategic foreign policy goals like trade and economic and military cooperation (Drager & Fidler, 2007). With up-to-date scientifically sound and evidence-based health advice, governments, businessmen, and diplomats must constantly strive to achieve the best health outcomes in the pursuit of foreign policy.

Diplomacy for science seeks to facilitate international cooperation, whether in the pursuit of top-down strategic priorities for research or bottom-up collaboration between individual scientists and researchers (Royal Society, 2010). When adapted to diplomacy for health, it entails facilitating international cooperation for health protection and promotion. The International Health Regulations of 2005 legally binding on all WHO members states whose purpose is to prevent, protect against, control, and provide public health response to the international spread of disease is an apt example of using diplomacy to achieve health goals.

Science for diplomacy draws on the attractivity and influence of the 'soft power' of science nationally and internationally. According to the Royal Society, science for diplomacy includes science cooperation agreements; new institutions to reflect the goals of science for diplomacy; educational scholarships; 'track two' diplomacy; science festivals and exhibitions. It basically falls within the scope of public diplomacy. When adapted to *health for diplomacy*, it entails the leveraging of health to promote foreign policy goals in cooperation agreements, designated organisations like the Pan American Health Organisation (PAHO), international health science scholarship, and international development for health among others.

THE EMERGENCE OF HEALTH DIPLOMACY AND THE CASE OF AFRICA

In 1902, the governments of the Americas met in Washington DC to establish the International Sanitary Bureau renamed the Pan American Sanitary Bureau (PASB) in 1923 (Howard-Jones, 1975). Known today as the Pan American Health Organisation (PAHO) is often considered to be the first known international health organisation in the world. Its roots can be traced back to 1889 when the first international conference of the American States was held in Washington attended by delegates from Brazil, Nicaragua, Peru, the United States, and Venezuela. Their interest was to seek methods of establishing and maintaining health regulations in trade between the various countries represented at the conference. The *Office International d'Hygiène Publique* (OIHP) followed in 1907 with an agreement of 12 countries (Belgium, Brazil, Egypt, France, Italy, the Netherlands, Portugal, Russia, Spain, Switzerland, the United Kingdom, and the United States). The membership of OIHP grew rapidly and in

1914 had reached 60 countries and colonies. The main concern was the prevention and control of infectious diseases by international quarantine. It required members to immediately notify if any outbreak of plague, cholera, yellow fever, typus, or smallpox was detected in any country. It was a precursor to the International Health Regulations.

Although American and European countries have sought to control cross-border infectious disease since the early fourteenth century (Loewenson et al., 2014), modern health diplomacy may be said to have emerged after the Second World War with the creation of the World Health Organization (WHO). The idea of the WHO, a specialised agency of the United Nations, was intended to promote health cooperation for peace and security between individuals and states. In the preamble, the State parties to the Constitution of WHO espoused the principles that the health of all peoples is essential to the attainment of peace and security and is dependent on the fullest cooperation of all (WHO, 1946). The constitution also acknowledges that unequal development in different countries in health care and especially communicable disease control is a common danger to all countries. The WHO was and remains the most ambitious multilateral effort at global health cooperation to date. Its membership has grown from 68 States at its creation in 1946 to 194 in 2021.

Another milestone in global health cooperation emerged with President Harry Truman who committed the USA to assist those countries and peoples he described as underdeveloped, by sharing the benefits of the progress the USA had achieved in science, technology, and industry to address misery, famine, and disease. The term 'underdeveloped' still in use today is often credited to Truman in 1949 (Haslam et al., 2009). From this conception of the world, the USA framed its foreign policy, not in terms of the old imperialist exploitation common with European powers but, in terms of fighting against global poverty viewed as a global threat to mankind. To operationalise this vision, the Agency for International Development (AID) was created in 1961 to administer the United States foreign aid program (Plano & Olton, 1969). Following in the path of the USA, the Development Assistance Committee (DAC) of the Organisation for Economic Cooperation and Development coined the term, Overseas Development Assistance (ODA) in 1969 to measure the value of development assistance from developed to underdeveloped countries. In 2015, the UN set the ODA target at 0.7 percent of GDP. A lot of ODA goes to social development in Africa notably in health protection and promotion. To facilitate the administration of ODA, many countries have set up special agencies to administer the international technical cooperation component of their foreign policies. Added to career diplomatic staff in Western embassies in Africa's capital cities, many international cooperation agencies have also seconded some of their staff to the continent where they are active in funding all sorts of development projects with health and its determinants featuring prominently in their activities. Table 2.1 captures the proportion of ODA as a percentage of all bilateral commitments of the top ten donors to Africa by sector in 2017. The assistance to the health sector and its determinant components occupies a respectful position in the proportion of total ODA flows to Africa. This is the same with assistance in the context of multilateral cooperation.

The DAC of the Organization for Economic Cooperation and Development (OECD) is not alone in fostering global health diplomacy. The African Union (AU) and the regional economic groupings in Africa have also positioned health cooperation as an essential component of security, trade, and prosperity on the continent. To achieve intra-African health cooperation, the AU has created specialised departments and agencies and encouraged the formation of regional groupings to foster cooperation for good health in African populations. The AU division of health, nutrition, and population aspires to forge a harmonised, concerted, and coordinated approach to health policy and health care delivery systems at the continental level (African Union Webmail, 2020 and AU, 2015). This is translated into similar aspirations at the regional groupings which also espouse the objective of harmonising health policies across their countries as a means of enhancing their capacities to control and prevent pandemics and epidemics; ensure food safety; and develop their pharmaceutical potentials, among others. This is true of the West African Health Organisation in ECOWAS; the Organisation for the Fight against Endemic Diseases in Central Africa (OCEAC) of the Economy and Monitory Commission of the Central African States (CEMAC); the East African Community Health Department in the East African Community (EAC); and the Protocol on Health in the Southern African Development Community (SADC).

The relevance of Global Health issues in Foreign Policy Analysis and practice was given further recognition and weight in 2007 by the Ministers of Foreign Affairs of Brazil, France, Indonesia, Norway, Senegal, South Africa, and Thailand when they issued what has become known as the Oslo Ministerial Declaration on Global Health. In their Declaration, the Ministers noted as follows:

In today's era of globalisation and interdependence, there is an urgent need to broaden the scope of foreign policy. Together, we face a number of pressing challenges that require concerted responses and collaborative efforts. We must encourage new ideas, seek, and develop new partnerships and mechanisms, and create new paradigms of cooperation. We believe that health is one of the most important, yet still broadly neglected, long-term foreign policy issues of our time ... It is generally acknowledged that threats to health may compromise a country's stability and security. We believe that health as a foreign policy issue needs a stronger strategic focus on the international agenda. We have therefore agreed to make an impact on health a point of departure and a defining lens that each of our countries will use to examine key elements of foreign policy and development strategies and to engage in a dialogue on how to deal with policy options from this perspective. As Ministers of Foreign Affairs, we will work to increase awareness of our common vulnerability in the face of health threats by bringing health issues more strongly into the arenas of foreign policy discussions and decisions, in order to strengthen our commitment to concerted action at the global level ... ensure that a higher priority is given to health in dealing with trade issues, and in conforming to the Doha principles, affirming the right of each country to make full use of TRIPS flexibilities in order to ensure universal access to medicines; strengthen the place of health measures in conflict and crisis management and in reconstruction efforts. (Ministers of Foreign Affairs of Brazil France Indonesia Norway Senegal South Africa and Thailand, 2007)

By ending the Declaration with an invitation to other Ministers of Foreign Affairs from all regions to join them in further exploring ways and means of attaining their objectives, it gave strong theoretical and political weight to the advocacy for the inclusion of health in foreign policy analysis.

Despite these admirable ambitions and goals, intra-Africa health diplomacy has remained in the shadows and doldrums of global health diplomacy. In a discussion brief of October 2015, the Regional Network for Equity in Health in East and Southern Africa (EQUINET), corroborates the discrepancy in health emergency responses between international and African agencies. In response to the West African Ebola Virus Disease (EVD) epidemic of 2014–2016, African sources contributed US$600 million (13 percent) of the total emergency funding of US$ 4558 million in May 2015 (EQUINET, 2015). This 13 percent included the US$ 1.2 million (0.03 percent) contributed by the African Union (AU, 2015). A similar trend occurred with the international response to COVID-19 dominated by the World Bank pledge of US$160 billion to more than 100 countries. Over US$50 billion of this amount was allocated to protect the poor and vulnerable people of Africa through health systems enhancement (World Bank, 2021).

As theoretically attractive as it may be, the political basis of health in foreign policy remains fragile and unattractive to the levers of power politics. While remaining sympathetic to its ideals, few countries around the world have translated that into concrete reality. There are few diplomatic missions in the world that distinctively have a position for the health attaché or counsellor. Despite this, no government can deny that health can be an instrument of foreign policy and that foreign policy serves health goals (Kickbush, 2006). These stands constitute the main basis of the rapidly growing literature on health and foreign policy. The UK and US governments now explicitly promote international health for global economic, financial, and political security. Between 2000 and 2016, the Bush and Obama administrations extended the frontiers of global health diplomacy starting with President's Emergency Plan for AIDS Relief (PEPFAR) initially set up by George W. Bush. This is arguably the largest ever global health intervention in terms of value by any single country in history. It has been renewed by subsequent US governments. Before leaving office in 2013, Hilary Clinton, Obama's first Secretary of State, created the Office of Global Health Diplomacy to respond to the US National Security and National Biodefense Strategies, which is built on the principle that halting and treating the disease at their points of origin is one of the best and most economical ways of saving and protecting American lives (US Department of State, 2022). Thus, US health diplomacy is essentially strategic.

'Investments in global health are a pillar of American leadership—advancing our national interests, making other countries more stable and the US more secure' (Obama administration). In concrete terms, US global health diplomacy brings the following strategic benefits to the country: goodwill so that countries collaborate with the US in attaining its strategic objectives; strengthening other economies turning them into viable trading partners; and building state capacity to produce stable countries, which all help to mitigate the chaos, war, and disruption.

References

AU Webmail. (2020). Division of Health, Nutrition and Population. African Union. https://au.int/en/sa/dhnp

AU. (2015). *Health, humanitarian affairs, and social development (HHS).* African Union. https://au.int/en/hhs

Davies, S. E., Elbe, S., Howell, A., & McInnes, C. (2014). Global health in international relations: Editor's introduction. *Review of International Studies, 40*(5), 852–834. https://doi.org/10.1017/S0260210514000308

Drager, N., & Fidler, D. P. (2007). Foreign policy, trade and health: At the cutting edge of global health diplomacy. *Bulletin of the World Health Organisation, 85*(3), 162. https://doi.org/10.2471/2FBLT.07.041079

EQUINET. (2015). *African responses to the 2014/2015 Ebola virus disease epidemic.* Discussion Brief. EQUINET. https://equinetafrica.org/sites/default/files/uploads/documents/EQUINET_GHD_Ebola_brief_Oct2015_for_web.pdf.

Felbaum, H., Lee, K., & Michaud, J. (2010). Global health and foreign policy. *Epidemiologic Reviews, 32*(1), 82–89. https://doi.org/10.1093/epirev/mxq006

Felbaum, H., & Michaud, J. (2010). Health diplomacy and the enduring relevance of foreign policy interests. *PLoS Medicine, 7*(4). https://doi.org/10.1371/2Fjournal.pmed.1000226

Fidler, D. P. (2005). *Health and foreign policy: A conceptual overview.* The Nuffield Trust.

Fidler, D. P. (2009). After the revolution: Global health politics in a time of economic crisis and threatening future trends. *Global Health Governance, 2*(2), 1–21. https://www.ghgj.org/Fidler_After%20the%20Revolution.pdf

Haslam, P. A., Schafer, J., & Beaudet, P. (2009). *Introduction to international development: Approaches, actors, and issues.* Oxford University Press.

Howard-Jones, N (1975). *The scientific background of the International Sanitary Conferences 1851–1938.* Geneva, World Health Organisation.

Koplan, J. P., Bond, T. C., Merson, M. H., Reddy, K. S., Rodriquez, M. H., Sewankambo, N. K., & Wasserheit, J. N. (2009). Towards a common definition of global health. *Lancet, 373*(9679), 1993–1995. https://doi.org/10.1016/S0140-6736(09)60332-9

Kickbush, I. (2006). The need for a European strategy on global health. *Scandinavian Journal of Public Health, 34*(6), 561–565. https://doi.org/10.1080/14034940600973059

Kickbusch, I., Lister, G., Told, M., & Drager, N. (2013). *Global health diplomacy: Concepts, issues, actors, instruments, fora and cases.* Springer.

Kickbusch, I. (2011). Global health diplomacy: How foreign policy can influence health. *British Medical Journal, 342*, d3154. https://doi.org/10.1136/bmj.d3154

Kickbusch, I., Silberschmidt, G., & Buss, P. (2007). Global health diplomacy: The need for new perspectives, strategic approaches and skills in global health. *Bulletin of the World Health Organisation, 85*(3), 230–232. https://doi.org/10.2471/BLT.06.039222

Kickbusch, I., Nikogosian, H., Kazatchkine, M. & Kökény, M. (2021). A guide to global health diplomacy: Better health-improved global solidarity-more equity. https://www.graduateinstitute.ch/sites/internet/files/2021-02/GHC-Guide.pdf

Kickbusch I. (2013). A game change in global health: the best is yet to come. *Public Health Rev., 35.* https://publichealthreviews.biomedcentral.com/articles/10.1007/BF03391687

Labonté, R. (2014). Health in all (foreign) policy: Challenges in achieving coherence. *Health Promotion International, 21*(S1). https://doi.org/10.1093/heapro/dau031

Labonté, R., & Gagnon, M. (2010). Framing health and diplomacy: Lessons for global health diplomacy. *Globalisation and Health, 6*(14). https://doi.org/10.1186/1744-8603-6-14

Loewenson, R., Modisenyane, M., & Pearcey, M. (2014). African perspectives in global health diplomacy. *Journal of Health Diplomacy..* https://www.tarsc.org/publications/documents/loewenson%20modisenyane%20pearcey_african%20perspectives%20in%20GHD.pdf

Macfarlane, S. B., Jacobs, M., & Kaaya, E. E. (2008). In the name of global health: Trends in academic institutions. *Journal of Public Health Policy, 29*(4), 383–401. https://doi.org/10.1057/jphp.2008.25

Ministers of Foreign Affairs of Brazil France Indonesia Norway Senegal South Africa And Thailand. (2007). Oslo Ministerial Declaration—Global health: A pressing foreign policy issue of our time. *Lancet, 369*(9570), 1373–1378. https://doi.org/10.1016/S0140-6736(07)60498-X

Nye, J. S., Jr. (2004). *Soft power: The means to succeed in world politics.* Public Affairs.

Plano J. C. & Olton R. (1969). The international relations dictionary. Holt Rinehart and Winston.

Royal Society. (2010, January 12). New frontiers in science diplomacy: Navigating the changing balance of power. *The Royal Society.* https://royalsociety.org/topics-policy/publications/2010/new-frontiers-science-diplomacy/.

UNGA. (2009). *Global health and foreign policy: Strategic opportunities and challenges—Note by the Secretary General.* A/64/365, United Nations.

UNSC. (2000). Resolution 1308 adopted by the Security Council at its 4172nd Meeting of 17 July 2000. S/RES/1308 (2000), United Nations.

US Department of State. (2022). The US Agency for International Department. Joint Strategic Plan, FY 2022–2026. https://www.usaid.gov/sites/default/files/2022-05/Final_State-USAID_FY_2022-2026_Joint_Strategic_Plan_29MAR2022.pdf

Smith, R., Fidler, D. P., & Lee, K. (2010). *Global health diplomacy research.* Trade, Foreign Policy, Diplomacy and Health Draft Working Paper Series, 1–18. *WHO Network on Global Health Diplomacy.*

World Bank. (2021, April 8). *World Bank's response to COVID-19 (Coronavirus) in Africa.* World Bank. https://www.worldbank.org/en/news/fact-sheet/2020/06/02/world-banks-response-to-covid-19-coronavirus-in-africa.

WHO. (1946). *Constitution of the World Health Organisation.* World Health Organisation. https://apps.who.int/gb/bd/PDF/bd47/EN/constitution-en.pdf?ua=1

CHAPTER 3

Health Diplomacy and Africa: An Overview

Zebulon Suifon Takwa

INTRODUCTION

The African wise saying that health is wealth and multitudes of related wisdom indicate the notion that the quest for the well-being of Africans by Africans has been part and parcel of the African aspiration from time immemorial. In addition, the ubuntu philosophy that 'you are because I am' is a further demonstration of what defines the relationships between many communities across Africa, thus underscoring the well-known adage that 'no nation is an island'. It is in this context that we have approached the understanding of the concept of health diplomacy in this chapter, with the conviction that it falls within the realm of the global village that the world has become. That we are emphasizing global health diplomacy is also an indication that it is lacking, inadequate or needs adjustments and innovations to ameliorate its current form.

This chapter discusses health diplomacy as an instrument of social justice and human rights in Africa, in the context of the global response to the COVID-19 pandemic, despite earlier initiatives such as the Millennium

Z. S. Takwa (✉)
United Nations Development Programme, Harare, Zimbabwe
e-mail: ztakwa@yahoo.fr

H. N. Ndi et al. (eds.), *Health Diplomacy in Africa*, Studies in
Diplomacy and International Relations,
https://doi.org/10.1007/978-3-031-41249-3_3

Development Goals (MDGs), the Sustainable Development Goals (SDGs), Trade-Related Aspects of Intellectual Property Rights (TRIPS), and many others. The Sustainable Development Goals (SDGs) adopted in 2015 were an affirmation of the global resolve to tackle social, environmental, and economic issues underpinning humanity and the planet by 2030. With the SDGs in mind, this chapter appraises the role of the African Union as an overarching structure and its Agenda 2063 as far as the issues of health are concerned. The chapter also overviews the multilateral and bilateral cooperation among member states, and how geopolitical interests have affected African states in their quest for equitable access to health care internationally.

The African Union's Agenda 2063 launched during the golden jubilee celebrations of the founding of the Organization of African Unity (OUA) is rooted in Pan-Africanism and African Renaissance and provides a robust framework for addressing past injustices and the realization of the twenty-first century as the African Century (African Union Commission, 2015a). Agenda 2063 is Africa's blueprint and master plan for transforming Africa into the global powerhouse of the future. It is the continent's strategic framework with the aim to revive the dream of Africa's founding fathers by achieving its goal for inclusive and sustainable development for unity, self-determination, freedom, progress, and collective prosperity of its people. For this to be realized, the citizens must be healthy enough and well-nourished, and adequate measures are undertaken to ensure access to quality healthcare services for all people.

The idea of health-for-all is not new. The slogan 'health for all by the year 2000' was one such resounding rhetoric that unfortunately ended without concrete results. Although Africa's health prospects are clouded with challenges such as COVID-19 and the abnormal behaviour of some powerful members of the international community, there are also silver linings and opportunities, which if addressed and harnessed, can significantly transform the health situation in Africa. This chapter will also briefly examine the challenge of the age-long brain drain of Africa's medical personnel and the resurgence of medical tourism where Africa's rich class patronize Western and Asian medical institutions. How the notion of people-centred health diplomacy can contribute to transforming these challenges into opportunities for a healthier and more prosperous Africa will be explored.

Finally, in attempting to address these puzzling issues, we posit that national ownership and innovations will be key in orchestrating a paradigm shift in the African health sector. The African diaspora, partnering with the private business sector and establishing horizontal partnerships in the framework of a renewed African solidarity drive, can be a game changer. Improved technology, the lessons from the COVID-19 pandemic, and the rise of nationalism, including vaccine nationalism at the detriment of Africa, should serve as a catalyst for Africa's awakening and mobilization.

THE AFRICAN UNION AND AFRICA'S HEALTH REAWAKENING AGENDA

With a population of about 1.3 billion, and projected population growth of 3.4–4 percent, extreme poverty remains persistently high in Africa. According to the World Health Organisation (WHO), Africa constitutes 25 per cent of the world's disease burden, while its share of global health expenditures is less than 1 percent. More than half of Africa's population is without access to essential health services and manufactures less than 2 percent of the modern medicine consumed in the continent (Chattu et al., 2021).

SDG 3 aims to ensure healthy lives and promote well-being for all, acknowledging good health as a universal and fundamental human right. The strategic role of health in the overall framework of sustainable development is not in doubt. SGDs such as 2, 6, 7, 8, 11, 12, 13, and 16 implicitly contain elements that have something to do with health. It is therefore imperative to reiterate that the implementation of the SDGs should be holistic and complementary. The interconnectedness transcends individuals, families, communities, institutions, and organizational levels. According to a public attitude survey of 36 African countries, inadequacies in Africa's health systems such as barriers to basic health services that include health facility shortages, inaccessible medical care, and poor governance for basic services strengthening remain evident (Wesonga & Kulohoma, 2020).

It is in the background of a challenging health context that the African Union in its Agenda 2063, Aspiration 1, envisions a 'Prosperous Africa based on inclusive growth and sustainable development'. To achieve this ambition, one of the key goals for Africa is to ensure that its citizens are healthy and well nourished, with commensurate investments made to expand access to quality healthcare services for all people. According to the Social Affairs Department of the Commission that promotes the work of the institution in health and nutrition, the AU works to ensure Africa develops and sustainably manages its health sector by putting in place the relevant sectoral institutions to support knowledge building as well as manage emergencies and disease outbreaks in the continent (African Union Commission, 2022). Africa draws these institutional and multilateral approaches from experiences and global best practices.

In the 1970s following the decade of political independence, most African governments embarked on long-term plans from 1975 to 2000 to address four main issues: (1) the development of human resources for health, (2) the promotion of environmental health, (3) control of communicable diseases, and (4) strengthening health services. In 1977, the World Health Assembly made the famous Health-For-All (HFA) Declaration as a health development policy objective and the adoption in Alma-Ata which positioned the primary health care approach as the strategy to attain the HFA. However, despite efforts by countries to prioritize primary health care as the framework for national health policies and plans, the global economic crisis and the subsequent structural adjustment plans jeopardized the efforts as other agendas soon took centre stage in the African region. However, although the Bamako Initiative of 1987 revived the concept of primary health care and emphasized more community participation, this was insufficient to regain the HFA desired progress (WHO Regional Bureau for Africa, 2000). In 1998 the World Health Assembly requested that its report, 'Health-For-All in the twenty-first century' (WHA 51,1998) becomes the framework for the development of future health policies. A World Health Assembly Declaration (WHA 51,71,998) was adopted, affirming the need to give effect to the 'Health-For-All in the twenty-first century' through the implementation of regional and national policies.

As one of Africa's initiatives towards addressing the long-term development objectives and challenges, the Lagos Plan of Action (1980–2000) was premised on the realization that Africa has been a major victim of the unfulfilled promises of global development strategies. As articulated in the Lagos Plan of Action that was enacted twenty years after independence, it was apparently clear that Africa was 'unable to point to any significant growth rate or satisfactory index of general well-being. Faced with this situation and determined to undertake measures for the basic restructuring of the economic base of our continent, we [Africa] resolved to adopt a far-reaching regional approach based primarily on collective self-reliance'. (OAU, 1980). The 1980 Lagos Plan of Action was a follow-up to the 'Monrovia Declaration of Commitment of the Heads of State and Government of the OAU on the guidelines and measures for national and collective self-reliance in economic and social development for the establishment of a new international economic order' in 1979. (ibid.). This new economy is still awaited today.

The link between health and nutrition is clear and therefore cannot be achieved without a commensurate focus on food security. In the post-independence era, particular importance was attached to addressing the deteriorating food and agriculture situation in the continent, as the food production and consumption per person were falling below the required nutritional levels. African countries had to resort to importing food, and this seriously drained the meagre foreign exchange resources and created constraints in financing development in Africa. The fundamental problem behind the food crisis in Africa was diagnosed to be the fact that few African countries concretely accorded due importance and priority to agriculture in terms of allocating adequate investment capital to the sector as well as giving sufficient attention to policies geared at raising productivity and improving the lives of the rural peasant farmers (OAU, 1980).

It was thus recommended that the development of agriculture should be undertaken in a holistic and integrated manner, taking into consideration other enabling factors in the context of an overall socio-economic development process. Moreover, in order to achieve an effective agricultural revolution in Africa, the necessity to involve the youth and halt rural-to-urban migration was invoked. As a matter of urgency, policies consistently emphasized the need not only to improve the living conditions on the farms but also to increase real incomes as a means of making agriculture more attractive and remunerative. The Lagos Plan of Action further called on all AU Member States to set up national strategic food reserves of the order of 10 percent of total food production, adopt coherent national food security policies (including the construction of storage facilities, creation of grain reserves, improvement of grain stock management, and better forecasting through the establishment of early warning systems); and to create a collective self-reliance mechanism through the establishment of sub-regional food security arrangements (OAU, 1980).

The Abuja Declaration (2001), a pledge by African Union countries to increase government health funding by at least 15 percent of the national budgets, remained a significant commitment to prioritize health above other priories that Africa is confronted with. Only a few African countries have been able to comply with this pledge. At the same time, the declaration urged donor countries to 'fulfil the yet-to-be-met target of 0.7 percent of their GNP as Overseas Development Assistance (ODA) to developing countries'. The average level of general government health expenditure from domestic resources (GGHE-FS) in African Union Countries was very close to US$10 with a thousand-fold difference between the minimum (US$0.38) and maximum (US$380). In terms of ODA, five of the 22 donors then reporting to the OECD were already giving at least 0.7 percent of their Gross National Income (GNI) with an average (unweighted) of 0.4 percent (OAU, 2001).

The Astana Declaration (2018) (Kazakhstan) was built on the Alma-Ata (USSR) Declaration (1978) and emphasized the importance of primary health care to address existing health challenges, renew political commitment to primary health care, and achieve universal health coverage. The Bali Declaration which amplified the Global Human Security Agenda in the Kampala Declaration (2008) remain largely unimplemented, due to budget constraints and weak political will.

With Africa's increasing disease burden, despite good plans and existing strategies, the African Union developed the Africa Health Strategy (AHS) 2007–2015 endorsed by the 3rd Conference of African Ministers of Health in 2007 and the 11th Session of the Ordinary Executive Council in 2008. The goal of the strategy was to enrich and complement Member States' efforts by adding value to existing health systems and structures using continental platforms. The AHS 2007–2015 provided strategic direction to Africa's efforts towards better health for all, drawing lessons from Africa's previous health goals attempts, including the MDGs. The AHS 2016–2030 adds value to Member States and Regional Economic Communities (RECs) health sector policy frameworks and strategies by its emphasis on addressing issues that reflect upstream strategic roles best suited for the African Union Commission and the RECs through which Member States can derive direct benefits such as economies of scale, collaborative efforts, and other advantages (African Union Commission, 2015b).

Agenda 2063 is expected to draw lessons from past plans and commitments. These include mobilization of the people and their ownership of continental programmes at the core; the principle of self-reliance and Africa financing its own development; the importance of capable, inclusive, and accountable governments and institutions at all levels and in all spheres, including health; the critical role of RECs as building blocks for continental unity; taking into account of the special challenges faced by vulnerable countries; and mutual accountability by citizens, governments, and institutions (African Union Commission, 2015, p. 1).

The AU's Africa Centre for Disease Control and Prevention (CDC) was set up as the lead institution to support African countries in promoting health and preventing disease outbreaks by improving prevention, detection, and response to public health threats. The Africa CDC seeks to strengthen Africa's public health institutions' capacities, capabilities, and partnerships to detect and respond quickly and effectively to disease threats and outbreaks, based on science, policy and data-driven interventions and programmes. Africa CDC plays a key role in linking various parties through the continental Event-Based Surveillance Unit (EBS), building the capacity of member States, field activities conducted through the Continental Emergency Operation Centre (EOC) as well as establishing Regional Collaborating Centres (RCC). The AU plans to launch a health volunteer corps within the Africa CDC. The African Volunteer Health Corps will be deployed during disease outbreaks and other health emergencies (African Union Commission, 2022).

The Vulnerable African Health Sector

Over the years, the African health sector had been under stress as result of the imbalance between resources and needs. Political instability has also contributed to the deterioration of health systems and services in terms of performance. Population growth has outsmarted economic growth, and the demand for goods and services in the health and education sectors has been abysmally inadequate. Many health problems are due to illiteracy and ignorance, and these have been aggravated by poor dietary and nutritional habits. Until the 1970s, the state was the sole guarantor of health in most African countries. This is no longer the case, especially since the advent of the structural adjustment programmes (SAPs) that saw African governments relinquishing most of their governance responsibilities, including health. The health sector suffered as it was deprived of resource allocation as the privatization experiment failed to be the answer to Africa's economic and social plight (WHO, Regional Bureau for Africa, 2000).

The WHO Regional Bureau for Africa 2000 in its 'Health for All policy for the 21st Century in the African Region: Agenda 2020' highlighted the obstacles to the effective implementation of health development programmes. These included health professionals' attitudes and resistance to change, unsatisfactory working conditions, imbalance in the distribution between personnel in urban and rural areas, and brain drain mainly due to inadequate remuneration and insecurity. Others include practices and customs that negatively affect health, inadequate disbursement of funds for full execution of budgets, misappropriation of funds, lack of complementary inputs, growing poverty, and limited political commitment to the development as an integral part of, and precondition for, socio-economic and human development (WHO Regional Bureau for Africa, 2000). The resurgence of insurgencies and internal wars in Africa and coup d'états have compounded the effective delivery of health services, including access to vulnerable populations.

The COVID-19 pandemic further exposed the prevalent weak health systems across Africa. Even the rich leadership class who had neglected the health sector while embarking on expensive health evacuation abroad were caught in their own trap of negligence. Borders (land, sea and air) were closed, and there was no room to escape the rot in the dilapidated health facilities in the countries. On the other hand, the resort to vaccine nationalism further exposed Africa's vulnerability to external influences as the continent depended almost exclusively on imports from abroad.

Prior to the pandemic, inequitable spending on health, as opposed to public spending, was the largest source of health financing in more than half of the African Union member states in 2017. According to experts, official development assistance still constitutes more than 20 percent of total health spending in 20 of the 55 African Union member states (ODI, n.d.). Despite the challenges confronting member states, more African countries are making progress and have significantly prioritized and financed their health sectors as a key emergency response as was witnessed during the COVID-19 and epidemics like the 2014 Ebola epidemic. It remains to be seen whether this is a shift in policy orientation, or it is just a short-lived development (ODI, n.d.).

A key lesson from the COVID-19 pandemic is that depriving the health sector of resources portends grave consequences for the entire economy, social dynamics, and politics, especially in Africa. In this regard, and as a way forward, there is a need to build a resilient health system as a safeguard against future pandemics. In addition, a focus on strong primary healthcare systems and a health-promotive capital that invests in the socioeconomic determinants by engaging with other related sectors is required. Third, investing in enablers like technology through partnerships with the private sector in global health diplomacy is recommended. According to the WHO Director-General, Tedros Adhanom Ghebreyesus, the issue of health financing is critical as voluntary prepaid health insurance policies tend to raise very limited funding. In some cases, it exacerbates inequalities and diverts scarce health human resources to serve the needs of the privileged wealthy than the poor (ODI, 2019). The thinking around insurance should therefore be universal coverage with adequate provisions of inclusivity to address the needs of the poor and vulnerable.

The AU emerged as the region that suffered most from the COVID-19 vaccine nationalism, as rich countries hoarded or restricted the sale of vaccines using various reasons to justify their 'nationalism'. This happened in a context where many, including Bill Gates, had predicted doom for Africa. While Bill Gates had predicted the pandemic could claim about 10 million lives in Africa, his wife then and co-chair of the Gates Foundation, Melinda Gates, added that without drastic actions, COVID-19 could lead to dead bodies littering the streets of Africa. On the contrary, Africa recorded fewer COVID-19 cases and deaths than many other parts of the world. Despite the poor quality of health systems across the African continent, the case fatality rates (CFR) on the continent remained among the lowest globally, hovering around 2 percent against Europe's 6.3 percent, South America's 3.4 percent, North America (3.9 percent), and a global CFR of 3.7 percent as of 7 August 2020 (WHO Health Policy Watch, 2020).

The decision by most African countries to quickly implement lockdown measures may have helped slow down the spread of the virus. However, widespread food insecurity and economic hardship forced many African countries to reopen their borders and economies, resulting in an increase in the spread of COVID-19. To ensure that the continent-wide systems are in place for the next pandemic and other health challenges, experts proffered the need for the AU to build on the leadership and governance that was demonstrated during the COVID-19 pandemic, ensuring effective processes, systems and structures and active engagement between the Commission and member states. Second, they emphasized the need for more joint action between the governments in repositioning health in terms of recovery efforts and domestic finance for health as propounded by the AU Declaration on the Africa Leadership Meeting: Investing in Health (ODI, 2019).

Another inspiration from the COVID-19 response in Africa has been the cooperation seen among various countries, and the coordination role being played by the African Center for Disease Control (Africa CDC). In the midst of the crisis, the Director of the Africa CDC, John Nkengasong ably coordinated access to testing kits and consumables including personal protective equipment for frontline health staff, capacity development and risk communication. Rwanda and other African countries like Ghana actively deployed innovative measures including robots to reduce contact of health workers with persons that tested positive as well as drones for the delivery of kits and medication to remote areas. Cashless transactions (mobile money) were also adopted to prevent possible transmission of the virus from one person to another through cash handling. The use of the iPad and mobile phone for collecting information, especially during contact tracing, was also another innovation. Many African countries saw the necessity to accelerate the decentralization of their health governance structures as part of their pandemic response efforts, including decentralized lab testing capacities, according to the WHO. (WHO Health Policy Watch, 2020).

MEDICAL TOURISM IN PERSPECTIVES

Medical tourism and the brain drain of Africa's medical personnel constitute a double tragedy for the continent. In September 2019, former Zimbabwean president Robert Mugabe died at a Singaporean Hospital. He was amongst a number of African leaders who leave their countries to seek medical treatment overseas. President Paul Biya of Cameroon has been a regular medical attendee in Switzerland during his more than 40 years in power. President Muhammadu Buhari frequently goes to the UK for a medical treatment which may last for months sometimes. The late Yar'Adua of Nigeria was following treatment in Saudi Arabia until he returned home and died in 2010. Ali Bongo, president of Gabon, suffered a stroke and was rushed to a hospital in Saudi Arabia in October 2018, while his father and predecessor, Omar Bongo died in Spain. Zambia's Levy Mwanawasa died in France, while Ethiopia's Prime Minister Meles Zenawi died in Belgium. The list of top political medical tourists is endless. The funds spent to treat top government officials abroad every year could build hundreds of first-class hospitals and medical facilities in Africa. In addition, leaders travel with elaborate entourages, and fly in expensive chartered and sometimes medicalised planes, including the cost of parking (Africa News, 2019). The national security implication of the presidential health tourists is humongous.

The example set by leaders has been emulated by the rich middle class in Africa, most of whom are civil servants using state resources to fund their travels abroad—mainly to Europe, North America, and Asia—for their medical needs. In 2016, Africans spent over $6 billion on outbound treatment. Interestingly, Africa has a billion-dollar medical tourism market and the involvement of African leaders through partnerships could be the key to accentuating it. Indian healthcare entrepreneurs and investors are already making significant moves to corner Africa's medical tourism market by establishing branches in the continent, especially in East Africa (Africa News, 2019). The opportunity for public-private initiatives to explore the potential of the promising health service industry is immense.

The Multi-Million Dollar African Medical Centre of Excellence (AMCE) currently under construction in Abuja, Nigeria, will contribute significantly to curtailing the current massive capital flight linked to medical trips abroad. The Federal Government of Nigeria and the African Export-Import Bank (Afreximbank) have signed the Host Country Agreement which will see the setting up of the 500-bed facility with an estimated cost of $750 million. The agreement was signed in September 2022 between the chairman of the Board of Directors of Afreximbank and the Nigerian Minister of Foreign Affairs. The AMCE Abuja is a first-of-its-kind quaternary-level medical facility in the African continent as a whole. It will promote Intra-African Trade medical tourism by offering a full spectrum of services in oncology, haematology, cardiology, and general healthcare across the continent, in addition to training, research and development capabilities. The AMCE Abuja will serve as the headquarters of other AMCEs to be launched across Africa (Vanguard Nigeria, 2020).

According to CNN, around 18,000 medical tourists are taking the trip over the Indian Ocean Island country to seek health treatment in hospitals in Mauritius. And the sector is growing, as heavy investments in infrastructure and human resources are underway to attract more foreigners, especially from Europe (particularly France) and Asia. Healthcare centres like *Centre de Chirurgie Esthetique* are capitalizing on the country's attractions—the beauty, luxury, and tranquillity—to locate hospital facilities near tourist attractions where visitors can experience a natural tourist feeling (CNN, 2018).

According to research, the effects of medical tourism in destination and departure countries are enormous. The practice of medical tourism can be seen as offering solutions to problems, with the potential to aid in the development of health care infrastructure in destination countries as it reduces the time spent waiting for medical appointments for residents of departure countries. It is also a revenue-generating industry, capable of generating revenues for destination countries as a form of health services trade. On the other hand, medical tourism is resulting in capital flights from departure countries. Some may still consider the practice as setting standards for health care. Due to low labour costs in destination countries, medical tourists may develop expectations of standards of human resource provision that are unaffordable, and therefore unattainable, in high-income departure countries (Johnston et al., 2010). However, the perception of better and more affordable medical services in some destinations in Asia has led to the infiltration of the profession by money-minded quacks. The lure of low cost has resulted in circumstances where desperate patients have been handled by unqualified professionals and end up paying more than what they were meant to pay. Most African families have been victims of this circumstance.

Overall, medical tourism remains a source of inequity, even as it brings financial benefits to the beneficiaries. Within destination countries, it can contribute to an internal brain drain of trained medical workers from rural to urban areas and from the public to the private sector. Medical tourists can face a significant drain on their own financial resources, and by engaging in travel abroad for medical services, they may contribute to a loss of impetus for reform of their home healthcare systems (Johnston et al., 2010). This syndrome is very much felt in Africa today. More studies on this subject will shed more light on the pros and cons of medical tourism. Notwithstanding, a glaring fact remains that the industry may grow at the detriment of the public sector health provision for ordinary people. COVID-19 came and the inability of the rich and political elite to be evacuated abroad brought some hard lessons and hope to the African public sector as leaders were caught in their own trap of negligence and everyone was compelled to use the same substandard medical facilities. Indeed, COVID-19 knew no social class.

HEALTH DIPLOMACY, THE NEW IMPERATIVE

South Africa is one example of an African country that has placed health discussions at the centre of its diplomacy of recent. When the Biden administration in early 2022 temporarily barred nearly all non-U.S. citizens who had visited South Africa and seven other southern African countries from entering the country following identification of the *Omicron* variant of COVID-19, many Africans denounced the move as 'travel apartheid'. President Ramaphosa qualified the travel bans as unjustified, unfair, and discriminatory. The Biden administration later reversed its stance and applauded South Africa for helping identify the Omicron variant as well as its efforts to produce domestic vaccines. With one of the best regulatory environments on the continent, South Africa made global headlines in February 2022, when researchers at Afrigen Biologics and Vaccines in Cape Town were able to reproduce the Moderna vaccine (The Africa Report, 2022).

As part of South Africa's health diplomatic efforts, Britain in November 2022 announced a new set of research collaborations with South Africa following President Ramaphosa's visit to the UK's Crick Institute, the biggest biomedical research facility in Europe, and Kew Gardens, with King Charles III's brother Edward. The British foreign minister James Cleverly stated that the partnerships, on areas such as vaccine manufacturing, genome sequencing and climate change, will 'benefit us all'. Britain has pledged to support genome sequencing at South Africa's National Institute for Communicable Diseases (NICD), which played a key role in detecting COVID-19 variants such as *Beta* and *Omicron*, in a push to improve antimicrobial resistance surveillance in Africa (Reuters, 2022).

Global health diplomacy entails a spectrum of issues ranging from health and health determinants to crucial foreign policy matters, including, national and international security, and trade. Kickbusch and Liu (2022) identify seven dimensions of global health diplomacy: negotiating to promote health in the face of other interests; establishing new governance mechanisms in support of health (like the Global Fund, the Vaccine Alliance); creating alliances in support of health outcomes; building and managing donor and stakeholder relations; responding to public health crises; improving relations between countries through health; and contributing to peace and security.

Diplomacy is part and parcel of the system of global health governance. Global health diplomacy was amply exemplified during the COVID-19 pandemic when multilateral cooperation was at its peak, with its attendant achievements and challenges, championed by the World Health Organisation (WHO). The imperative for global diplomacy in response to the COVID-19 pandemic, the biggest since the 1918 influenza pandemic, in a joined-up response between countries with hitherto strained relations confirmed what the Director-General alluded to when he said: 'no one is safe until everyone is safe' (Kickbusch & Liu, 2022). Issues of geopolitical interests, nationalism and weak institutions were at the core of the diplomacy of COVID-19 diplomacy.

The diplomatic standoff between the USA and China brought a stalemate at the WHO, the UN Security Council, the Group of 20 (G20) and the Group of Seven (G7). The only unique multilateral agreement on health security adopted in 2005—the International Health Regulations (IHRs)—failed to hold ground, and many countries failed to fulfil their obligations, closed borders, and blocked the export of critical medical supplies. The WHO was powerless and lacked the resources to match the exigencies of the time. Even the declaration of COVID-19 as a public health emergency was politicized and delayed (Lancet 2020; 399:2156–66). The Access to COVID-19 Tools (ACT) accelerator was established, through the COVID-19 Vaccines Global Access (COVAX) initiative, as the means to speed up development, production, and equitable access to COVID-19 test kits, treatment, and vaccines across the globe, but the high-income countries (HICs) ignored the initiative and embarked on vaccine nationalism practices, deploying huge amounts of money to secure exclusive access to vaccines for their populations and their allies (Kickbusch & Liu, 2022; 399:2156–66).

While the COVAX initiative aimed at establishing solidarity for humanity and equity, other nations were out to reinforce their geopolitical advantage (Kickbusch, 2021). Africa found itself at the periphery of this power game, and this does not only raise an ethical concern but also a moral one. This brings to the fore critical issues that underlie international relations, such as the Trade-Related Aspects of Intellectual Property Rights (TRIPS) and the ability of African countries to procure essential and life-saving drugs for their healthcare delivery systems drawing from the HIV-AIDS and the COVID-19 pandemics. There is a need for African countries to leverage the AU as well as individual countries like South Africa in exploiting the flexibilities in the TRIPS to enhance the continent's pharmaceutical capacities in the case of epidemics and pandemics such as Ebola virus diseases, HIV/AIDS, and cholera. The AU and African governments need to institutionalize a robust campaign and advocacy to lessen the grip of the TRIPS instrument on essential drug production or procurement in Africa. It is perhaps in this context that the World Trade Organization (WTO) Director-General, Ngozi Okonjo-Iweala, stated that the health of populations is also the business of the WTO, adding that trade contributes to public health and the WTO can be in the forefront of assisting member states access vaccines and medical supplies (Kickbusch & Liu, 2022; 399:2156–66). She was indeed pleading with the African cause.

It should be recalled the Okonjo-Iweala, before becoming the WTO head, was one of the 4 African Union's Special Envoys, alongside Donald Kaberuka, Tidjane Thiam and Trevor appointed by the President of the Republic of South Africa, Cyril Ramaphosa in his capacity as the then AU Chair of Heads of State (2020–2021), to mobilise international support for Africa's efforts to address the economic challenges African countries will face as a result of the COVID-19 pandemic. The Special Envoys will be tasked with soliciting rapid and concrete support as pledged by the G20, the European Union and other international financial institutions (African Union, 2020).

Addressing complex global health challenges requires concerted and multifaceted multi-actor diplomacy that includes nonstate actors (informal sectors, non-governmental organizations, civil society organizations, academia and most especially, the private sector). This was very much highlighted in the *Paris Declaration on Aid Effectiveness* in the context of highly asymmetrical donor-recipient power relations and the high dependency on health assistance amongst African and developing countries.

The donors also have a dilemma when it comes to deciding how best to engage with recipient countries with regard to health assistance. One such platform for multilateral cooperation is the International Health Partnership (IHP), which serves as an example of a development approach to global health policy. The IHP+ was equivocal over whether it will deliver more health aid or only improve the efficiency and effectiveness of what is currently on offer. Launched in September 2007, with leadership from the UK and Norway, the IHP+ intended to operationalize the *Paris Declaration on Aid Effectiveness* within the health sector. The *Paris Declaration* emphasizes the 'harmonization' of activities by donors and external agencies, following increased bilateral health aid and independent global health initiatives following criticisms that such an approach is weakening recipient countries' capacities to develop their own comprehensive health system plans. The UK was one of the few countries that advocated the pooling of resources by 'international development agencies to directly finance the budgets of health sector plans in developing countries (UKHG), to ensure country ownership and sustained and predictable donor funding' (Labonte & Gagnon, 2010). This is the format that African countries like Rwanda have been advocating for – direct budget support.

Though political and economic issues tend to drive the wedge between competing nations, trans-frontier health epidemics and pandemics naturally entail collective approaches in dealing with the threats. For Africa to fully assume its role as an important member of the global community, her numerical might and prowess must begin to be deployed (particularly the youthfulness of its population), economic assets (vast mineral deposits) and its renewable energy potentials leveraged to negotiate a better deal. The rich African biodiversity in the Congo Basin and beyond, and the untapped African pharmacopoeia are some of the opportunities for Africa's medical future. The rules of classical diplomacy, which many African countries met at the banquet table, may need to be revised as 'the continent of the future' begins to assert itself. The new international order that may emerge must be anchored on a win-win basis (Loewenson et al., 2014). However, this idealism must be taken with caution. The Russian-Ukraine war and the resurfacing of the cold war rhetoric and mentality may undermine the hopes already raised. The rise of the BRICS (Brazil, Russia, India, China, and South Africa) alongside G7, and G20 platforms may be an opportunity as it may pose challenges to the status quo. Africa must capitalize on the current dynamics and cease to be a like a helpless, bedridden patient, swallowing any tablet offered in a typical beggar-having-no-choice posture.

The Ebola virus spread and the challenge it posed remains a major health concern. In 2022, countries like the Democratic Republic of the Congo (DRC) and Uganda are still battling with Ebola, a few years after West Africa (Sierra Leone, Liberia, Guinea, and Nigeria) was hit by the deadly virus. There was the impression by Africans that the rest of the world did not respond appropriately because the disease was localized in Africa. Ironically, the spread of the virus had its own 'diplomatic bearings' following the incident in July 2014 where a Liberian diplomat entered Nigeria and brought the virus into the country, causing a diplomatic embarrassment and uproar. Patrick Sawyer who brought the Ebola virus into Nigeria had possibly contracted the virus from his late sister and was unfortunately cleared to travel to Nigeria for a conference organised by the Economic Community of West African States. Nigerians blamed the Liberian Government for the oversight although Nigeria's Health Minister, Onyebuchi Chukwu, later confirmed that the Liberian government had apologized for the incident, noting that Nigeria was free of Ebola Virus until its importation by the Liberian American. Mr Sawyer's action placed unnecessary stress on Nigeria's health system (Ibekwe, 2014). Incidentally, it was also an Italian traveller who was tracked and traced as the first conveyor of COVID-19 to Nigeria (Vanguard Nigeria, 2020).

OPPORTUNITIES AND WAYS FORWARD

The African Continental Free Trade Area (AfCFTA) which was launched in January 2021 provides a unique opportunity for trade, including medical facilities if Africa succeeds in manufacturing to connect its 1.3 billion population in the 54 countries of the continent. This will also facilitate the effective curbing of the importation of fake drugs that remain a serious health menace to the continent. The AfCFTA will promote and consolidate intra-African trade, continental industrialization, and production of its own medicine, in addition to the enhancement of South-South cooperation.

The African forest and savanna that have provided the source of healing for the continent's populations for centuries are yet to be fully explored and transformed for health, economic and environmental benefits. Cultivating medicinal plants is a huge economic prospect for Africa (Halilu, 2022). Traditional African medicine (what is also called alternative medicine) that has been despised or undermined remains a source of hope if Africa can draw lessons from the Asian countries, including India that have patented almost all medicinal plants in their forests. Protecting and securing African forests that have been subject to abusive logging activities of timber companies is key to biodiversity conservation. This will also directly contribute to the fight against climate change as forests constitute the much-needed carbon sinks that regulate ozone layer depletion.

The thousands of African medical personnel who have migrated to greener pastures in the Middle East and in Western countries can play an important role in investing in knowledge, expertise exchange and giving back to their communities. Their knowledge, networks of contacts and experiences are critical for the African renewal. African countries must also prioritize health and enhance the motivation packages of medical doctors. A situation where rank-and-file soldiers earn more than medical doctors is unacceptable for countries that value the health of their citizens and the critical importance of medical doctors and other health workers. The mass exodus of nurses trained in developing countries but recruited in developed countries is a phenomenon that must be checked because of its negative consequences on health services in Africa.

African solidarity is very critical for a breakthrough in lobbying for Africa to take its rightful place in the comity of nations by seeking the equity and well-being of its citizens. The African Solidarity Initiative (ASI) was launched during the 19th Ordinary session of the Summit of Heads of State and Government of the AU in July 2012, with the view to mobilizing enhanced support from within the continent for post-conflict reconstruction and development in countries emerging from conflict. The objective of the ASI was to promote African solidarity, mutual assistance and regional integration, and propel the continent to a higher level of development and self-confidence, driven by the motto: 'Africa helping Africa'. The ASI was a major innovation and fruit of the AU's years of experience that has enabled the Commission at large, to practically bring on board an authentic African contribution to post-conflict reconstruction discourse/practice (ASI, 2020). Today's solidarity for the prevention of pandemics, epidemics and communicable diseases remains an imperative for Africa.

The idea of African solidarity was at the crux of the liberation struggle for independence. So far, political independence was secured. What is left is economic independence and building the required solidarity around health issues through collective diplomacy and engagement is crucial. The legal basis for expanding this solidarity is anchored on the AU's 'Inter-African Convention establishing an African Technical Cooperation Programme' adopted during the Kampala OAU summit in 1975. Article 1 (b) of the convention on aims and objectives of the programme emphasizes the quest to facilitate the comparison of scientific and technological knowledge as well as of experiments and experience relating to development among African countries (OAU, 1975). National ownership of the efforts, decentralization of health structures right to the communities, and the popular participation of the masses are critical (UNECA, 2010).

While we advocate for multilateralism and cooperation in addressing the world health and food insecurity challenges through diplomacy, it is important to draw attention to the resurgence of new threats to global peace. The Russia-Ukraine conflict has ignited the fear of the return of the Cold War rhetoric, suspicion, and mistrust, with Africa at the receiving end again. Voting patterns become yardsticks for sanctions and rewards, including food and health by some western powers. This will further undermine global efforts at addressing common challenges as geostrategic interests will undermine the march towards sustainable development. Nevertheless, the Russia-Ukraine crisis can be an opportunity for Africa to look inwards and reduce its dependency on the outside world by producing a larger portion of what it consumes.

CONCLUSION

Fondly called 'the continent of the future', and rightly so, the twenty-second century is Africa's. Most African countries attained independence during the 1960s and are just about 60 years old. With a rapidly growing population, there is a need to reap the demographic dividends of the youthful population for the continent's economic transformation. However, Africa is not a country. The complexity of dealing with 55 different entities with their peculiarities and challenges, some due to the hangovers of European colonization, the existence of the African Union and the rapidly evolving regional economic communities (RECs) and regional mechanisms, is a great opportunity. The lessons from its precursor, the OAU and the Agenda 2063 remain a great vision for the future of the continent. Health and food security in Africa must cease to be a slogan. The capacities and the capabilities are legions. Crafting the right approaches for renewed diplomacy on health on a win-win basis remains a task that current and future generations of Africans must embark on.

Africa's diaspora can draw inspiration from the Chinese, Indians and other Asian and Latin American countries that became agents and pillars for the socio-economic leap forward their countries have experienced. The African diaspora that the AU has elevated to a full region in its regional arrangements is a demonstration of the political will to recognize an untapped asset. National processes necessary to translate these options into concrete acts are needed, including the contentious issues of double nationality that some African countries still abhor for political rather than economic reasons. A paradigm shift is needed for win-win African diplomacy to deploy economic lenses in seeking agreements and signing conventions, including health-related ones because health is wealth. These agreements will also have to include those for transborder peace and security because where war advances, diplomacy including soft power retreats.

REFERENCES

Africa News. (2019, March 10). Africa's health tourism presidents. *Africa News.*. https://www.africanews.com/2019/10/03/africa-s-health-tourism-presidents-travel/.

African Union. (2020). https://au.int/en/pressreleases/20200412/african-union-chair-president-cyril-ramaphosa-appoints-special-envoys

African Union Commission. (2015a). Agenda 2063: The Africa we want. African Union. https://au.int/en/agenda2063/overview.

African Union Commission. (2015b). *Africa Health Strategy 2016–2030*. Addis Ababa, Department of Social Affairs.

African Union Commission. (2022). Accessed October 3, 2022. https://au.int/en/promoting-health-nutrition

ASI. (2020). Reinvigorating the African Solidarity Initiative for robust implementation of the African Union's Post-Conflict Reconstruction and Development Policy. https://www.accord.org.za/conflict-trends/reinvigorating-the-african-solidarity-initiative-for-robust-implementation-of-the-african-unions-post-conflict-reconstruction-and-development-policy/.

Chattu V. K., Knight, W. A., Adisesh, A, Yaya, S., Reddy, K. S., Di Ruggiero, E., Aginam, O., Aslanyan, G., Clarke, M., Massoud, M. R., & Jha, A. (2021). Politics of disease control in Africa and the critical role of global health diplomacy: A systematic review. *Health Promotion Perspectives.* 11(1), 20–31. https://doi.org/10.34172/2Fhpp.2021.04.

CNN. (2018, January 29). Mauritius offers medical care in the midst of pleasure. *Marketplace Africa.* https://edition.cnn.com/2018/01/29/africa/mauritius-investing-big-medical-tourism/index.html

Halilu, E. M. (2022). Cultivation and conservation of African medicinal plants for pharmaceutical research and socio-economic development. In K. Sanjeet (Ed.), *Medicinal Plants.* IntechOpen.

Ibekwe, N. (2014, August 12). How Liberian government cleared Patrick Sawyer to travel to Nigeria while under observation for Ebola. Premium Times https://www.premiumtimesng.com/investigationspecial-reports/166560-exclusive-how-liberian-govt-cleared-patrick-sawyer-to-travel-to-nigeria-while-under-observation-for-ebola.html

Johnston, R., Crooks, V. A., Snyder, J., & Kingsbury, P. (2010). What is known about the effects of medical tourism in destination and departure countries? A scoping review. *International Journal for Equity in Health, 9,* 24. https://doi.org/10.1186/1475-9276-9-24

Kickbusch, I. (2021). The new geopolitics of global health. *Global Solutions Journal, 7,* 50–56. https://www.global-solutions-initiative.org/wp-content/uploads/2021/05/Global-Solutions-Journal-7-Summit-2021-Edition.pdf

Kickbusch, I., & Liu, A. (2022). Global health diplomacy-reconstructing power and governance. *The Lancet, 399*(10341), 2156–2166. https://doi.org/10.1016/S0140-6736(22)00583-9

Labonte, R., & Gagnon, M. (2010). Framing health and foreign policy: Lessons for global health diplomacy. *Globalization and Health, 6*(14). https://doi.org/10.1186/1744-8603-6-14

Loewenson, R., Modisenyane, M., Pearcey, M. (2014). African perspectives in global health diplomacy. *Journal of Health* Diplomacy online. https://www.

tarsc.org/publications/documents/loewenson%20modisenyane%20pearcey_african%20perspectives%20in%20GHD.pdf.

OAU. (1975, August 01). Inter-African convention establishing an African Technical Cooperation Programme. *African Union.* https://au.int/en/treaties/inter-african-convention-establishing-african-technical-co-operation-programme.

OAU. (1980). *Lagos plan of action for the economic development of Africa, 1980–2000.* AU Printing Press.

ODI. (2019). 12 leaders' perspectives on supporting Africa's health systems through Covid-19. https://odi.org/en/insights/12-leaders-perspectives-on-supporting-africas-health-systems-through-covid-19/.

ODI. (n.d.). https://odi.org/en/insights/12-leaders-perspectives-on-supporting-africas-health-systems-through-covid-19/

Organization of African Unity (OAU). (2001). "Abuja Declaration on HIV-AIDS, Tuberculosis and other related Infectious Diseases", African Summit on HIV/AIDS, Tuberculosis and Other Related Infectious Diseases, Abuja, Nigeria, 24-27 April 2001 (OAU/SPS/ABUJA/3).

Reuters (2022, November 2023). Britain and South Africa agree health partnership on second day of state visit. https://www.reuters.com/world/uk/britain-south-africa-agree-health-partnership-second-day-state-visit-2022-11-23/

The Africa Report. (2022). https://www.theafricareport.com/238241/south-africa-five-things-on-the-agenda-for-president-ramaphosas-visit-to-the-white-house/?utm_source=newsletter_tar_daily&utm_campaign=newsletter_tar_daily_06_09_2022&utm_medium=email&utm_content=edito_full_story

UNECA. (2010). Popular participation and decentralization in Africa, UNECA Press. https://archive.uneca.org/sites/default/files/PublicationFiles/popular-participation-decentralization-in-africa.pdf.

Vanguard Nigeria. (2020). https://www.vanguardngr.com/2020/02/coronavirus-how-italian-imported-disease-into-nigeria/

Wesonga, C. A., & Kulohoma, B. (2020). Prioritising health system to achieve SDGs in Africa: A review of scientific evidence. In M. Ramutsindela & Mickler, D. (Eds.), *Africa and the Sustainable Development Goals,* SDG Series, Springer. https://doi.org/10.1007/978-3-030-14857-7_11.

WHO-Regional Bureau for Africa. (2000). "Health-For-All Policy for the 21st Century in the Africa Region: Agenda 2020", Fiftieth Session, Ouagadougou, Burkina Faso, 28 August-2 September 2000, (AFR/RC50/8 Rev.1), 21 August 2000.

CHAPTER 4

The Role of Regional Agencies in African Health Diplomacy

Anna Baninla Mbur Tasha and Guy Elessa

INTRODUCTION

The outbreak of COVID-19 in the Chinese city of Wuhan in late 2019 and its exponential global spread has been an unprecedented event for the modern world. The medium of contamination seemed to have followed the most usual route; the international travel route, the fastest being airports and aeroplanes. In a few weeks, the whole world was under pressure and deaths from the COVID-19 virus. Although the pandemic created left desolate economic and social scars in many countries, it helped to expose entrenched global social inequalities that exist among nations, continents, and peoples. The effects of the COVID-19 pandemic are a strong justification for concerted action by states in preventing, controlling, and managing global health problems through cooperation and diplomacy. For instance, during this pandemic, rather than cooperate on joint plans to

A. B. M. Tasha (✉)
High Commission for the Republic of Cameroon, London, UK

G. Elessa
Cameroon Embassy, Paris, France

© The Author(s), under exclusive license to Springer Nature Switzerland AG 2023
H. N. Ndi et al. (eds.), *Health Diplomacy in Africa*, Studies in Diplomacy and International Relations,
https://doi.org/10.1007/978-3-031-41249-3_4

57

share expertise and increase the global availability of medical equipment, there were export bans, equipment poaching, and *beggar-thy-neighbour* bidding wars. Rather than cooperate to develop a vaccine together, 'vaccine nationalism' took centre stage, with countries unilaterally pursuing independent research programmes, and even attempting to pull research skills from other countries. This *'my country first'* attitude has become a global movement—and has undermined the will and capacity of different countries to respond effectively to emergencies like COVID-19 (Brown & Sisskund, 2020).

Few African countries have strong health systems. Consequently, approximately 1.6 million Africans died of malaria, tuberculosis, and HIV-related illnesses in 2015. These diseases can be prevented or treated with timely intervention and enhanced access to appropriate and affordable medicines, vaccines, and other health services. But less than 2 percent of drugs consumed in Africa are produced on the continent, meaning the health system relies heavily on expensive imported drugs affordable to only a few privileged ones. Without access to medicines, Africans are vulnerable to the three big killer diseases: malaria, tuberculosis, and HIV/AIDS. Globally, 50 percent of children under the age of five (5) years who die of pneumonia, diarrhoea, measles, HIV, tuberculosis, and malaria are found in Africa (Pheage, 2017).

Modern international health cooperation dates back nineteenth century when the French Government initiated the organisation of 14 International Sanitary Conferences in Europe and North America between 1851 and 1938 to standardise international quarantine rules against cholera, plague, and yellow fever (Howard-Jones, 1975). From a focus on multilateral cooperation, the concept of global health diplomacy has also included independent states' initiatives for preventing the spread of infectious diseases in third countries. As an emerging field of foreign policy, health diplomacy has been defined as a practice that meets the 'dual goals' of improving both global health and international relations (Valenza, 2020).

The uniquely high disease burden of the African continent compared with the rest of the globe begs the point for African countries to invest their scarce resources in strengthening their health systems through skills training and investments in pharmaceuticals to ensure the provision of affordable essential drugs to its populations. Intra-African health diplomacy and collaboration are indispensable here because the continent must face its own problems directly. This chapter examines the contributions of African regional and sub-regional groupings to health cooperation and its inherent challenges. This chapter will therefore tackle the role of African sub-regional groupings in addressing health challenges on the African continent through Health Diplomacy.

Africa's Health Diplomacy Actors

State Actors

Among the State or institutional actors, are the Heads of State and Ministers of Health. The Heads of State provide the general orientation. The ministries of health elaborate the national health policies and strategies, which are often defined and shaped in consideration of the broader international health environment which may change over time. In doing so, they work in collaboration with the foreign affairs ministries for the implementation of foreign policies. Both ministerial departments work with the assistance of their embassies accredited to foreign countries in implementing the country's foreign policy objectives. Ambassadors and their staffs assume all functions as directed by the sending State. Traditionally, embassies dealt mainly with the strategic interests of their states which covered political, economic and commercial, cultural, military, and consular cooperation affairs. Lately, with the recognition of the strategic importance of international health to state security, several embassies have opened the office of health attachés.

The Health Attaché is a relatively new concept in the field of diplomacy and in embassies. They are now seen as playing a key role in diplomacy as they are responsible for promoting or facilitating cooperation between countries in the sector of health. This function has been mainly reserved for persons who have primarily worked as medical practitioners for embassies staff. In the United States, for example, health attachés work with the US Government, multinational organisations, non-state actors, and the host country government (Kelly, 2021) to promote suitable health policies in their respective countries.

Non-State Actors: Intergovernmental Organisations

The UNO is the largest intergovernmental organisation in the world. Its affiliated organs such as the World Health Organisation (WHO) and the United Nations International Children's Emergency Fund (UNICEF) are veritable platforms of multilateral health diplomacy. Other UN agencies whose mandates have health policy implications are the United Nations High Commission for Refugees (UNHCR), the United Nations Development Programme (UNDP), and the World Bank. In times of crisis, the WHO plays an important resource mobilisation role for developing countries and is a main actor in health system reforms in Africa (Gupta, 2021). In 2014, the WHO was a central player in coordinating technical support to the fight against the Ebola outbreak in West Africa (WHO, 2015; Kaner & Schaack, 2016). In 2018, UNICEF warned that the Ebola virus disease (EVD) was becoming endemic in the Great Lakes region of the Congo Basin and could not be addressed by humanitarian actors alone. It coordinated a participatory response to the virus by working with the local people on their preparedness and response in Uganda, South Sudan, Burundi, and Rwanda. They have supported people at risk in communication and community engagement, to inform, protect, and engage the influential community and religious leaders on the dangers of EVD. They have also educated people on prevention and control and have provided psychological support to families, particularly affected by the disease (UNICEF, 2019). Very recently in Central Africa, UNICEF launched World Immunisation Week in celebrating vaccine heroes who promote the use of vaccines to protect every child against diseases in West and Central Africa and whose passion and engagement have made both routine and COVID-19 vaccination possible (UNICEF, 2022).

Both UNICEF and the WHO work very closely with national governments to improve water, sanitation, and hygiene (WASH); infection prevention control (IPC); and healthcare services. Such multilateral actions are necessary, significant, and important for public health interventions as they are associated with a reduction in the transmission of preventable infections (Munos & Zaid, 2022). These two organisations not only work with governments but also with other intergovernmental organisations in Africa notably the African Union (AU) and its regional economic communities (RECs).

Non-State Actors: International Non-Governmental Organisations

Religious organisations, international humanitarian organisations, and development nongovernmental organisations (NGOs) and groups also play an important role in shaping health cooperation by being implementation and feedback channels of international health policies. Doctors without Borders, Catholic Relief Services, the International Red Cross and Red Crescent Movement, The Human Relief Foundation, the pan-African Global Alliance for Chronic Diseases, the Planetary Health Alliance, the Global Health Network, or the Global Fund to Fight AIDS, Tuberculosis and Malaria are all international NGOs that work with African governments to create a platform for negotiating and implementing global health policies and services.

Non-State Actors: Multinational Corporations (MNC)

Multinational corporations (MNCs) have become very important actors in international health. This group may be the most controversial of all because their goals and policies are profit-oriented and exclusively mercantilist. In this respect, MNCs invest in health services as a corporate social responsibility to the populations in the catchment areas of their activities. Corporate social responsibility in health and other social components of life enables corporations and companies to be socially accountable to stakeholders, the public, and the communities in which they operate (Fernando, 2022). Corporate social responsibility is sometimes considered the most effective cooperation or collaboration for the creation of positive social change in Africa.

THE AFRICAN UNION (AU) HEALTH STRATEGY: EXAMINING THE AFRICA CENTRE FOR DISEASE CONTROL (CDC)

According to Agenda 2063 of the AU, the organisation hopes to ensure that Africans are healthy and well nourished, with adequate levels of investments that are made to expand access to quality healthcare services for all people. The African Union works to ensure Africa develops sustainably by promoting—nutrition and health.

The AU Health and Nutrition Policies and Strategies

The African Health Strategy 2016–2030 (AHS 2016–2030) and the Africa Region Nutrition Strategy (ARNS) for the period 2015–2025 are entwined because nutrition is an important determinant of health. The latter identifies the potential role of the AU and the AU Commission (AUC) in the elimination of hunger and malnutrition. It is based on the

AU's 2014–2017 Strategic Plan and reflects the recently initiated AU Agenda 2063, which articulates the longer term vision of the continent (African Union Commission, 2015). The strategy aims to provide guidance to a systematic and consistent effort to eliminate the problems of hunger and malnutrition across all AU Member States. It also details the specific role and tasks that the AUC and its implementing agencies (including RECs) and partners will undertake to lead and support the implementation process of the strategy according to their respective mandates and capacities. To improve nutrition levels on the continent, the AU has worked with member states on specific activities like the Cost of Hunger in Africa Study (COHA), which has improved knowledge about the social and economic impact of child undernutrition on the continent and the interventions that countries need to make to address and remedy the issues identified as contributing to poor nutrition (AU, n.d.). All of these apply in the context of 'prevention is better than cure' and the commitment of the AU to address major health challenges in Africa.

Agenda 2063—*The Africa We Want* and the 2030 Agenda for Sustainable Development, including its Sustainable Development Goals. Other policy frameworks from which AHS 2016–2030 is reinforced include the Sexual and Reproductive Health and Rights Continental Policy Framework and its revised Maputo Plan of Action 2016–2030, the Pharmaceutical Manufacturing Plan for Africa (PMPA), the African Regional Nutrition Strategy 2015–2025 (ARNS), the various AU Abuja commitments aimed at combating AIDS, tuberculosis, and malaria in Africa, the Catalytic Framework to End AIDS, TB and Eliminate Malaria in Africa by 2030 as well as the Global Strategy for Women's, Children's and Adolescent's Health (2016–2030) (Department of Social Affairs, 2015).

The AHS 2016–2030 provides strategic direction to AU member states in their efforts to create better-performing health sectors and recognises existing continental commitments while addressing key challenges in efforts to reduce the continent's burden of disease, mainly by drawing on lessons learned and taking advantage of the existing opportunities. Its strategic directions require multi-sectoral collaboration and adequate resources with leadership to champion its implementation and ensure effective accountability for its results (ibid.).

Another dimension of multi-country collaboration is through the strengthening of South-South as well as South–North–South partnerships, which support the health sector. Based on past experiences the 'codes of conduct', which seek to influence the recruitment of African health workers by industrialised countries can also help channel the benefits of the African diaspora to impact the health sector positively. This includes utilising African Diaspora technological and financial assets that can be linked to key gaps in health financing, knowledge, technology, or service capacity. Some innovative financial and technological advances among African diasporas have succeeded in adding value to African health cooperation, including telemedicine, research, and development of new drugs and health technologies (Department of Social Affairs, 2015).

The African Centre for Diseases Control and Prevention (Africa CDC)

The idea for the creation of the Africa Centres for Disease Control and Prevention (Africa CDC) came up in 2013 after one of the most devastating outbreaks of the Ebola Virus Disease. It was eventually established in 2017 during the 26th Ordinary session of the Heads of State and Governments of the AU. Its guiding principles are leadership, credibility, ownership, delegated authority, timely dissemination of information, transparency, accountability, and value addition (Statutes of the Africa Centre for Disease Control and Prevention 2016). Article 3, of the Statutes, states that one of the main objectives of the *Africa CDC is the promotion of partnerships and collaborations among member States to address emerging and endemic diseases and public health emergencies.*

The agency thus focuses on supporting the public health initiatives of member states and strengthens the capacity of their public health institutions to detect, prevent, control, and respond quickly and effectively to disease threats. The Africa CDC has centres in each of the five (5) subregions of Africa: Egypt for North Africa, Gabon for Central Africa, Kenya for East Africa, Nigeria for West Africa, and Zambia for Southern Africa. These centres work directly with member states to implement the Africa CDC's strategy through public health surveillance and virtual communities of practice. They have succeeded to provide responses to some of the issues related to Lassa fever, Meningitis, and Monkey Pox in Nigeria. The Africa CDC has also been presented to address health problems related to the plague in Madagascar and Cholera in Ethiopia, as well as the Ebola Virus Disease in the Democratic Republic of the Congo.

This structure receives support in medical epidemiology training from the United States of America CDC. In July 2022, the Africa CDC also received a $100 million grant from the World Bank to strengthen Africa's preparedness and response capabilities to health emergencies (AU/Africa CDC, 2022). In response to the Ebola Virus Disease in the DRC, the Africa CDC has been able to:

(a) Activate its Emergency Operation Centre (EOC) to support national outbreak response efforts.
(b) Mobilise its Epidemic Response Team (ERT) for imminent deployment—the team is comprised of experts with previous experience in epidemic response specifically dealing with the Ebola outbreak in West Africa in 2014 and in the DCR in 2017.
(c) Set aside USD$ 250,000, for outbreak response activities, whilst more resources are mobilised (Africa CDC, 2018).

CHALLENGES OF HEALTH DIPLOMACY IN THE AU AND AFRICA CDC

Despite the innovations in the institutional framework of the African Union, there seems to be a latent trend within the organisation's incapacity to act and pursue Africa's health interests and strategy independently. In the same vein, the Africa CDC has shown its incapacity to maintain functional and operational independence. They have also shown shortcomings in their ability to mobilise continental financing to respond to major crises facing the African continent. Most of the finances for the organisation have come from international partners such as WHO, UNICEF, the United States, and the World Bank among many others.

The Africa CDC and all its related mechanisms (the *African Event-Based Surveillance Unit*, the *Continental Emergency Operation Centre*, and the *Regional Collaborating Centres*) have been put in place to support individual countries achieve successful responses to disease control and prevention. Despite their efforts, these mechanisms have not yet demonstrated their ability to enforce health cooperation among member states. Among some of the most important challenges for the AU, and Africa CDC is the achievement of greater regional and collective competence in defining and implementing a common health policy for Africa's sub-regions and mobilising the necessary resources from within the continent.

The Africa Health Strategy 2016–2030 surprisingly did not belabour the role of African sub-regional economic groupings in the implementation of the said strategy. It states that '*Regional Economic Communities will provide technical support to Member States, advocate for increased resources for health systems strengthening, harmonize the implementation of national Action Plans, monitor and report progress, identify and share best practices*'.

The Role of African Sub-Regional Groupings in Health Diplomacy

The activities of the following RECs: Arab Maghreb Union (AMU), the Common Market for Eastern and Southern Africa (COMESA), the East African Community (EAC), the Economic Community of Central African States (ECCAS), the Economic Community of West African States (ECOWAS), and the Southern African Development Community (SADC) are informative about the role each of them plays in the implementation of health diplomacy in Africa.

The Arab Maghreb Union (AMU)

The Arab Maghreb Union (AMU) was founded in February 1989 in Marrakesh. At the time the treaty was approved, the member states agreed to coordinate, harmonise, and rationalise their policies and strategies to achieve sustainable development in all sectors of human activities. In addition to the treaty, the Marrakesh Summit adopted the solemn declaration on the establishment of AMU and its work program. The Union's objectives were defined as strengthening the ties of brotherhood which link the member states and their peoples to one another; achieving progress and prosperity for their societies and defending their rights; contributing to the preservation of peace based on justice and equity; pursuing a common policy in different domains; and working gradually towards achieving the free movement of persons and transfer of services, goods, and capital among them (United Nations Economic Commission for Africa, 2016).

Despite their aim to pursue a common policy in different domains, the member countries of the AMU seem not to have considered health as a major component of their cooperation. This is evident with the institutions put in place by the treaty of Marrakesh. The AMU has the following institutions: the Presidential Council; the Council of Foreign Affairs Ministers; the Follow-Up Committee for Union Affairs (each member appointing one member of its government into the Committee); and the Specialised Ministerial Committees composed of economy and finance, infrastructure, food security, and human resources. There is no ministerial committee for health.

This notwithstanding, North African countries have invested significantly in public health services since the 1970s. According to the UN Economic Commission for Africa, investments in medical insurance, vaccination, access to water and better nutrition have resulted in lower infant and maternal mortality, longer life expectancy, and increased labour productivity. Algeria, Libya, and Tunisia are among the 20 countries that recorded the biggest leap in the Human Development Index between 1990 and 2012. These countries have adopted cross-sectoral approaches to get increased benefits from health, education, and potable water initiatives at an opportune time of demographic transition. However, health care in the Maghreb region also suffers from many weaknesses, including inefficient management, deteriorating quality and unsustainable funding in the public health services, low coverage of low-income and unregistered workers, regional disparities in public health coverage and quality, and poor regulation and supervision of private healthcare providers (Larbi & Lars, 2017). For example, because of the narrow health insurance coverage (restricted to employees in the formal sector) in countries like Morocco and Mauritania, access to basic health care is very low among the uninsured population. Their out-of-pocket payments for health services are among the highest in developing countries.

Moreover, recent studies show increasing pathologies in most Maghreb countries.[1] Obesity has emerged as a healthcare issue in the Maghreb, driven by changes in consumption and lifestyle brought about by higher incomes. Similarly, as the region's population ages, pathologies such as cancer, hypertension, and diabetes are becoming more common. HIV/AIDS has also emerged as a key concern. Meanwhile, in Tunisia and to a certain extent Morocco, health services have the potential to become a major export sector and could thus contribute to the economic objective of job creation and inclusive growth (ibid.).

The Common Market for Eastern and Southern Africa (COMESA)
The history of COMESA began in December 1994 when it was formed to replace the former Preferential Trade Area (PTA), which had existed from

[1] ibid.

the earlier days of 1981. COMESA (as defined by its Treaty) was established '*as an organisation of free independent sovereign states which agreed to co-operate in developing their natural and human resources for the good of all their people*' and as such it has a wide-ranging series of objectives which necessarily include in its priorities the promotion of peace and security in the region. With 21 member states; a population of over 583 million; a gross domestic product of $805 billion; a global export/import trade in goods worth US$ 324 billion, COMESA forms a major marketplace for both internal and external trading in Africa.

Like AMU, COMESA did not factor health in its sub-regional diplomacy. Nonetheless, following the outbreak of the COVID-19 pandemic, it decided to integrate health cooperation into its functioning and operations. Ministers responsible for health from the COMESA region have adopted rules of procedure to guide the establishment of a COMESA health desk and a regional statutory committee on health matters. This follows the recommendations of the 42nd COMESA Council of Ministers meeting held in November 2021 which decided that a committee on health should be established (COMESA, 2022). The set-up of the structure is ongoing, even though there has been a COMESA Health Framework for 2016–2030 to investigate the health problems of the Community (COMESA Health Framework, 2016). The newly adopted draft rules of procedure have been discussed and reviewed by health experts in consultation with other Regional Economic Communities and partners such as the Africa CDC. Specifically, the COMESA Health Desk is expected to facilitate the development of a sub-regional policy and strategic framework on health, promote and coordinate the implementation of health programmes, promote research and sharing of best practices on health, promote local manufacturing of medicines, prepare reports, and service meetings of member states (COMESA, 2022).

The East African Community (EAC)
The East Africa Community is one of the fastest-growing sub-regional groupings in Sub-Saharan Africa. Its annual GDP growth rate was 6.2 percent in 2015. The region witnessed a dramatic increase in life expectancy from 51 years in 2005 to 61 years in 2016; a progress that comes with new challenges of the growing burden of non-communicable diseases such as high blood pressure, diabetes, and cancers. Yet, the burden of communicable diseases such as HIV/AIDS, malaria, and tuberculosis;

maternal, neonatal, and nutritional diseases and injuries have remained stubbornly high in the sub-region (East Africa Community, 2018).

Further, the increasing global health security threats of epidemics, pandemics, and antimicrobial resistance threatens the integrity of the region's health systems. Health insurance coverage ranges from less than 2 percent in Uganda and South Sudan; to 25 percent in Tanzania; 28 percent in Kenya; 50 percent in Burundi; and 92 percent in Rwanda. About 70 percent of the EAC's medicines, vaccines, and other health technologies are sourced from outside the region. Achieving universal health coverage (UHC) is an ambitious sustainable development target whose attainment is heavily dependent on the symbiotic relationship between health, cooperation, and economic development.

Undertaking joint action towards the prevention and control of communicable and non-communicable diseases, and control pandemics and epidemics of communicable and vector-borne diseases that might endanger the health and welfare of the residents of the community and cooperate in facilitating mass immunisation and other public health community campaigns, the response to such a regional epidemiological emergency could be complex and may involve national, regional, and international agencies. An efficient and quick flow of information across borders is, therefore, crucial for averting such incidents of cross-border spread. The re-establishment of the EAC in 1999 provides room for increased collaboration in disease surveillance and epidemic control and prevention of spread (EAC, 2022).

To promote the achievement of the objectives with respect to cooperation in identified priority health activities in the East African Sub-region, as set out in the EAC treaty, five standing technical working groups are responsible for handling detailed health matters. These are medicines and food safety; control and prevention of sexually transmitted infections (STIs), HIV and AIDS; Control and Prevention of Communicable and Non-Communicable Diseases; Health Research; Policy and Health Systems Development; and, Reproductive, Child, Adolescent Health and Nutrition. For the implementation of the health-related objectives of the EAC, the East African Health Research Commission (EAHRC) saw the day to oversee success in their health diplomacy approach.

The East African Health Research Commission (EAHRC)

The EAHRC is a mechanism for making available to the EAC, advice on all matters of health and health-related research and findings that are necessary for knowledge generation, technological development, policy formulation, and practice. It is the principal advisory institution to the EAC on Health Research and Development. The Mission of the EAHRC is to improve the health and well-being of citizens of the Community by generating, accessing, capturing, assessing, synthesising, disseminating, and utilising health research and findings, as well as technological development that is suitable and relevant to the Community and its people (EA Health, 2022).

The Research Commission is the principal advisory institution to the Community on all matters related to health, research, and development. The functions of the Research Commission include ensuring the development of comprehensive networks for research linking member institutions; promoting collaborative health research programmes; promoting the exchange and dissemination of health research information through conferences, workshops, publications, use of ICTs, and other media; playing a critical advocacy role and search for research grants and required resources; promoting community outreach activities in the implementation of research findings; promoting the application of knowledge from research to strengthening regional health policy and practice; and facilitating the development of regional health policies and their implementation (ibid). Amidst other objectives, the EAHRC has developed a strategic regional initiative that incorporates different programmes to tackle the health problems in the region. Some of the programmes include:

- The Young East African Health Research Scientists' Forum (YEARS' Forum), an initiative to empower the next generation of research scientists and leaders in East Africa to be able to shape the future of health.
- East African Government Leaders, Legislators, and Legal Executives Forum (EAGLES Forum) which brings together EAC government leaders, members of parliament, officials from the judiciary, health experts, and the EAHRC to discuss health issues, pertaining to the sub-region.
- The East African Health and Scientific Conference (EAHSC), an EAC biennial event convened in East Africa by the EAHRC in col-

laboration with a host EAC Partner States. Hosting the event is rotational to each of the Partner States and is coordinated through the ministries responsible for EAC affairs, ministries responsible for health and other relevant organisations.

- The Official East African Web Portal for Health Information: www. eahealth.org is the official comprehensive compendium of health information in East Africa. It provides information on the regional health sector and of each of the Partner States.
- The EAHRC Journals
  - *East African Health Research Journal:* contains peer-reviewed articles, original articles, reviews, book reviews, short communications, surveys, commentaries, opinions on policy or practice, essays, and reports from East Africa.
  - *East Africa Science:* publishes scientific research and innovation in health including clinical trials (on investigational medicinal products, devices, and diagnostics), application of health technologies and solutions, and other related matters.
- The Regional East African Community Health Policy Making and Implementation (REACH PMI) initiative addresses the 'know-do gap' through a structured and proactive approach to apply the available evidence, knowledge, and best practices.
- The Regional East African Community Health Research Funding and Accessing (REACH RFA) initiative aims at identifying research priorities for health, mobilising resources, managing the resource, and conducting regular and thorough monitoring and evaluation of the impact of the resource and outputs to the health and well-being of the citizens.
- East Africa Health Cloud is a regional, real-time central data store for capturing, storing, retrieving, analysing, and managing national and regional health data.
- East African Cross-Border Health Services Pilot Programme: The populations that live along the EAC borders face health challenges that are unique to cross-border areas and can best be addressed collectively through an EAC regional initiative.
- The EAHRC has established or facilitated the establishment of regional networks of research, academic, and other health-related organisations to address priority regional health agendas. The insti-

tutions have teamed up with international reputable academic institutions to allow for knowledge and technology transfer and sharing.
These networks support the translation of health research into policy
in East Africa. Some of the networks are as follows:

- East African TWENDE Clinical Trials Network (acronym:
  TWENDE-CTN): The word *Twende* comes from the Eastern
  African lingua franca, Swahili which means 'encouraging each
  other to move forward together'. TWENDE's broad objective is
  to create a network of complementary Centres of Excellence in
  the East African Community region, develop a critical mass of
  personnel, technology, and infrastructure to perform the
  *International Conference on Harmonisation and Good Clinical
  Practice* (ICH-GCP) standard clinical trials.
- Holistic Approach to Unravel Antibacterial Resistance in East
  Africa (HATUA). Hatua is a Swahili word synonymous to 'take
  action'. The consortium is established with the broad objective of
  providing a coordinated regional response to curtail the imminent
  impact of antimicrobial resistance. Embedded within the EAC
  Partner States, HATUA takes the global antimicrobial resistance
  crisis in a regional holistic context and uses a range of research
  approaches from clinical, microbiological, and geographical to
  modelling and social sciences, to identify, understand, and map
  the burden and drivers of antibiotic resistance across different
  communities and environments in East Africa (EA Health, 2022)

The East African Community is one of the most operational sub-
regional groupings in Africa. Their structures are operational with diverse
programmes and initiatives. The major challenge they may face is developing a 100 percent mobilisation of funds from within the Community or
Africa and a good benchmark for other African sub-regional groupings.

THE ECONOMIC COMMUNITY OF CENTRAL AFRICAN STATES (ECCAS)

The Economic Community of Central African States was established on
October 1983 by members of the Economic and Monetary Community
of Central Africa (CEMAC), São Tomé and Principe, and members of the

Economic Community of the Great Lakes Countries (DRC, Burundi, and Rwanda). ECCAS was, however, inactive for several years due to financial constraints, conflicts in the Great Lakes area, as well as the war in the Democratic Republic of Congo where some member states (Rwanda and Angola) were proxies. Nevertheless, in October 1999, ECCAS was formally designated into the African Economic Community as one of the eight pillars of the African Union (UNECA, n.d.).

Article 60 (2) of the Treaty instituting the ECCAS stipulates that member states shall use their human resources fully and rationally to initiate sub-regional cooperation in public health, medical research, traditional medicine and pharmacy, and the exchanges of experiences.

Equipped with a Directorate of Health, the Community of Central African States has underscored the importance of setting up a regional health coordination structure in Central Africa—the Organization for Health in Central African Sub-region (OHCA) which member states had committed to creating since 2011. The new leadership of the ECCAS Commission is intent on speeding up implementing this long-standing ECCAS Decision. Setting up its regional health organisation will allow the Commission to coordinate member country's responses to epidemics/pandemics, as well as to other health issues in the sub-region. To date, a tripartite WHO-Africa CDC and ECCAS commission has been formed to support this process (Ngandu, 2021).

However, as a contribution to the response to COVID-19, various ECCAS organs were mobilised for the development of a Regional Response Plan. In March 2020, the ECCAS Commission developed a holistic multi-sectoral situational analysis paper on the impact of COVID-19 on cross-cutting issues, as well as a COVID-19 response strategy against the pandemic, which revolves around the following four strategic axes: prevention of the transmission; deaths or case management; mitigating the social, economic, and security effects associated with COVID-19; and preventing cross-border transmission.

The Convening of the ECCAS Ministerial Meeting on Health, on 24 June 2020, which allowed for the establishment of a common and effective strategy for dealing with the COVID-19 pandemic, is a sign that this sub-region is ready to develop health collaboration (ibid.).

The adoption of the sub-regional pandemic response strategy on 30 July 2020, as well as the regional pandemic surveillance, has prompted the ECCAS Commission to deploy its technical support teams to the Republic of Angola and the DRC.

A major challenge for ECCAS' health diplomacy is the urgent need to finalise the establishment of a Central African health organisation for the formulation and management of health policies and their implementation, in collaboration with the member states. It would also be useful for ECCAS authorities to benchmark the East African Community and the EAHRC to consider best practices or they could learn from the ECOWAS which has also attained a considerable level of success in health diplomacy.

THE ECONOMIC COMMUNITY OF WEST AFRICAN STATES (ECOWAS)

The Heads of State and Government of fifteen West African Countries established the Economic Community of West African States (ECOWAS) on 28 May 1975 in Lagos, Nigeria. They were Benin, Burkina Faso, Côte d'Ivoire, The Gambia, Ghana, Guinea, Guinea Bissau, Liberia, Mali, Mauritania, Niger, Nigeria, Sierra Leone, Sénégal, and Togo. ECOWAS is considered one of the pillars and fast growing African Economic Community.

The West African sub-region has a population of about 357 million (about 1/4 of Africa's population). The importance of health protection and disease control and prevention led ECOWAS to set up the West African Health Organisation (WAHO) in 1987. It is the regional agency responsible for safeguarding the health of the people in ECOWAS. This is done through the initiation and harmonisation of the policies of member states, the pooling of resources, and cooperation with one another, for collective and strategic combat against the health problems of the sub-region. WAHO has transcended linguistic borders and hurdles in the sub-region to serve all fifteen ECOWAS Member States. The WAHO protocol grants it the status of a specialised agency of ECOWAS.

WAHO is a proactive instrument of regional health integration that enables high-impact and cost-effective interventions and programmes by maintaining sustainable partnerships; strengthening capacity building; collecting, interpreting, and disseminating health information; promoting cooperation and ensuring coordination and advocacy among member states, and exploiting information communication technologies for the attainment of its objectives. Through its strategic programmes, WAHO has undertaken measures to combat malaria, malnutrition, HIV/AIDS, and maternal and infant mortality; improve access to medicines and vaccines, encouraged epidemiological surveillance, as well as training and health information management in the sub-region.

The ECOWAS Assembly of Health Ministers oversees the work of WAHO. The challenges that require multinational collaboration include epidemics, the trade in counterfeit medication, and the harmonisation of policies to address common health problems. The development of health research in the sub-region forms the basis for using evidence to bring about improvements in health systems and to address some of these challenges. Thus, research is of paramount importance for WAHO to achieve its mandate (Aidam & Sombie, 2016).

The National Health Research System (NHRS) has been defined by WHO as a system that provides the governance, development of research capacities, knowledge generation, and evidence utilisation mechanisms, as well as the accompanying sustainable financing mechanisms of any country's health system for the conduct of its health research activities. The NHRS is an important component of any modern health system and defines the environment in which health research is nurtured and performed. NHRSs have been found to be weak in many regions across Africa. WAHO's initial strategic plan (2003–2007) did not take the enormity of this weakness into account and thus did not focus specifically on research, but rather on the diseases of greatest burden in the sub-region. However, a second WAHO strategic plan (2009–2013) was developed in consultation with development partners and covered the broader areas of WAHO's institutional development, coordination and harmonisation of policies, health information, promotion and dissemination of best practices, development of human resources for health, medicines and vaccines, development of traditional medicine, diversification of health financing mechanisms, and the development of research (Aidam & Sombie, 2016).

Analysing the health situation in the ECOWAS sub-region in 2019, WAHO identified the most common health problems that were declared health concerns in the ECOWAS space. These were Lassa fever, cholera, measles, poliomyelitis, meningitis, dengue fever, anthrax, and Crimean-Congo haemorrhagic fever (WAHO, 2019). That same year the outbreak of COVID-19 hit the world. In response to the pandemic, WAHO quickly involved the sub-regional Health Ministries, national public health institutions, and partners by distributing a weekly sensitisation epidemiological bulletin from January 2020. It initiated weekly online meetings with National Public Health Institutes (NPHI) directors as well as directors of national laboratory services to discuss situational updates, challenges, and the needs of each country. Still, with COVID-19, WAHO worked closely with member states and held joint press briefings. The most memorable was held by the Director General of WAHO, Stanley OKOLO, with the Nigerian Minister of State for Health, Olurunnimbe MARORA, on 17 February 2020, when they announced that the WHO had declared the COVID-19 outbreak a 'public health emergency of international concern' (Herpolsheimer, 2022). The WAHO staff also worked closely with member states of ECOWAS towards strengthening airport surveillance, especially with direct flights to or from China. Working with the Africa CDC, WAHO supported the increased capacity of regional reference testing laboratories dedicated to testing COVID-19.

With regard to the Ebola Virus outbreak in West Africa in earlier 2014, neighbouring countries first adopted protectionist measures by closing their borders with Guinea, Liberia, and Sierra Leone. Some African airline companies shut down their flight connections with Ebola-affected countries. The West African Health Organisation (WAHO) was the first to hold an expert committee meeting on Ebola and its impact on the region. Ebola was a top agenda item for all ECOWAS Heads of State summits and Health Ministerial and Defence chiefs' meetings. On 10 July 2014, ECOWAS leaders decided to set up a regional solidarity fund to raise money for a regional Ebola response. Nigeria contributed US$ 3 million, Guinea US$ 500,000), Liberia (US$ 500,000), Sierra Leone (US$ 500,000), and WAHO (US$ 500,000) and to the ECOWAS Pool Fund for Ebola (USD 1 million). The Government of Ghana offered the WHO and international a logistics hub for the dissemination of medical equipment in the sub-region. On September 25, the *West African Economic and Monetary Union* Commission also granted a subsidy of 60 million CFA francs (EUR 0.9 million) to each of its member countries, to boost preventive measures (SWAC Club Secretariat, OECD , 2014).

WAHO's collaboration with foreign partners and donors such as the European Union (EU) and the German International Cooperation Agency (GIZ Gmbh) launched the 'Support to the Regional Centre for Surveillance and Disease Control in the ECOWAS Zone' project, which aimed at preventing a reoccurrence of the Ebola Virus Disease epidemic in the sub-region. Co-financed by the EU and GIZ with 4 million and 12 million Euros, respectively, the project is for a two-year term and will support members to improve communication on health risks due to infectious diseases; inter-institutional coordination and communication; human resources in the field of disease control and digital surveillance systems; and management of epidemics.[2]

The major challenge the ECOWAS will have to overcome is the financing of WAHO's functioning and operations within the West African sub-region. Together with the East African Community and the East African Health Research Commission, the West African Health Organisation should become benchmarking organisations from which all other African sub-regions will need to find inspiration from.

The Southern African Development Community (SADC)

As Southern Africa strives to enhance its economic growth, the health of its citizens remains paramount in ensuring a sustainable future. One of the objectives of SADC is to achieve an acceptable standard of health for all citizens. This goal derives from the SADC health programme, developed in 1997, in line with global and regional health declarations and targets. Three key policy documents have been developed to underpin the implementation of the programme:

- The Health Policy Framework;
- The SADC Protocol on Health, and
- The Regional Indicative Strategic Development Plan.

The SADC Health Policy plans to raise the regional standard of health for all citizens to an acceptable level, by promoting, coordinating, and supporting efforts of member states to improve access to high-impact health interventions. This framework was developed by the SADC Health Ministers and approved by the Community's Council of Ministers in September 2000. It proposes policies, strategies, and priorities in the areas of health research and surveillance; health information systems; health promotion and education; HIV and AIDS and sexually transmitted diseases; communicable and non-communicable disease control; disabilities; reproductive health; health human resources development; nutrition and food safety; and violence and substance abuse (SADC, 2022).

Article 3 of the SADC Protocol on health addresses the objectives of the organisation and stipulates that '*State Parties shall cooperate in*

---

[2] "EU, ECOWAS, GIZ Launch Regional Support to Improve Surveillance and Response Networks against Epidemics in the West African Region", www.eeas.europa.eu.

addressing Health problems and challenges facing them through effective regional collaboration and mutual support under this Protocol, for the purposes of achieving the following objectives:

(a) *to identify, promote, coordinate, and support those activities that have the potential to improve the health of the population within the region.*

(b) *to coordinate regional efforts on epidemic preparedness, mapping, prevention, control, and where possible the eradication of communicable and non-communicable diseases.*

(c) *to promote and coordinate the development, education, training, and effective utilisation of health personnel and facilities.*

(d) *to facilitate the establishment of a mechanism for the referral of patients for tertiary care.*

(e) *to foster cooperation and coordination in the area of health with international organisations and cooperating partners.*

(f) *to promote and coordinate laboratory services in the area of health, to develop common strategies, and to address the health needs of women, children, and other vulnerable groups.*

(g) *to progressively achieve equivalence and harmonisation and standardisation in the provision of health services in the region; and*

(h) *to collaborate and cooperate with other relevant SADC sectors*

SADC member states are responsible for financing their own health budgets. There is no specific SADC organisational budget for health policy as implementation follows a bottom-up approach. The SADC Secretariat develops relevant regional protocols with funds from SADC member states and donors. In 2013, external funding in SADC amounted to US$67,600,000 for a total of 58 projects. The Regional Indicative Strategic Development Plan (RISDP) is said to emulate EU policies of integration and development and is determined by the material dependence of SADC on the EU. As such, donors and governments work together to develop SADC-specific policies and protocols. At this stage in SADC's development, donor aid seems essential for sustaining regional health policies and systems strengthening (Penfold & Fourie, 2015).

Some of the SADC health policies, plans, and strategies that have been implemented and are still running within national health programmes include the Maseru Declaration on the fight against HIV and AIDS (2003); the SADC Draft Strategic Plan for the Control of Tuberculosis (2007–2015); the SADC HIV and AIDS Strategic Plan (2010–2015); the

SADC Malaria Elimination Framework (2010); the SADC Malaria Strategic Framework (2007–2015); the SADC Minimum Standards for the Prevention, Treatment and Management of Tuberculosis (2013–2017); the SADC Pharmaceutical Business Plan (2007–2013); the SADC Regional Minimum Standards for the prevention of Mother to Child Transmission of HIV (2009); the SADC Regional Minimum Standards for the Prevention, Treatment and Management of Malaria (2010); the SADC Sexual and Reproductive Health Business Plan (2011–2015); the SADC Strategic Framework for Control of Tuberculosis in the SADC Region (2012); the Sexual and Reproductive Health for SADC (2006–2015); The Draft Declaration on Tuberculosis in the Mining Sector (2012); The Health Policy Framework (2003); The Minimum Standards for HIV Testing and Counselling (2009); The Regional Indicative Strategic Development Plan (2001); and The SADC Minimum Standards for Child and Adolescent HIV, TB and Malaria Continuum of Care (2012) (Penfold & Fourie, 2015).

With the outbreak of the COVID-19 pandemic, SADC ministers of health agreed to harmonise and coordinate their efforts to respond to the virus in the region. However, levels of preparedness vary considerably among SADC countries, due to their individual national health policies. Nonetheless, the WHO regional office for Africa worked with member states to address gaps in prevention, impact mitigation, and other intervention with emergency and contingency funds. Ten of the sixteen SADC member states also agreed to share information on the COVID-19 outbreak (WHO, African Region, 2020).

The SADC Health Protocol allows for each country to run its own individual country health policy depending on the health challenges facing the sub-region or each of the countries. The sub-region officials and member states may want to consider optimising their cooperation, as the situation of the COVID-19 did impose by the creation of a sub-regional organisation like WAHO in ECOWAS to facilitate and coordinate cooperation work and responses to health problems in Southern Africa.

CONCLUSION AND RECOMMENDATIONS

Global health has emerged over the past decade as a new form of diplomacy within the context of shifting donor–recipient relationships. Novel types of health alliances and the rise of 'south-south' cooperation are important because health crises like the Ebola in West and Central Africa,

HIV/AIDS, and the novel coronavirus (COVID-19) pose fundamental challenges to the resiliency of regional and continental health strategies. Health diplomacy complicates the understanding of diplomacy because it extends into new spaces with diverse actors and manifold forms of negotiation. It is multilevel, including 'core diplomacy' with high-level interstate negotiations over health (notably within the WHO) and 'multi-stakeholder diplomacy', where various bilateral and multilateral organisations work with national governments to develop, implement, and monitor national and regional health initiatives (Anderson, 2018).

In Africa, regional health diplomacy has helped establish a US$200 million new health financing initiative to achieve UHC across the continent's 54 countries. The high cost of drugs and medical supplies is one of the significant hindrances to health care in Africa. To overcome this problem, a number of initiatives are being implemented—The Pooled Procurement agreement signed by seven small African Island States in 2020 (Cabo Verde, Comoros, Madagascar, Mauritius, São Tomé and Príncipe, and Seychelles) aims at reducing the cost and improving access to high-quality medicines (Chattu et al., 2021; WHO, 2019). The African Medicine Agency (AMA) and Partnerships for African Vaccine Manufacturing (PAVM) are worthy of mention here.

It is worth noting that intra-African health diplomacy is small, limited, imbalanced, and volatile. There is an urgent need to build on Africa's potential to achieve sustainable growth and cooperation in the health sector. Coordination and collaboration among African countries is essential to address the problems related to health, disease control, and prevention. Some of these problems could be summarised as follows:

- The absence of health coordination agencies in all the sub-regions and Regional Economic Communities affiliated with the African Union makes it difficult to harmonise health policies and tackle major health problems with adequate resources. Some of the sub-regions have already developed fully operational agencies that promote health research and respond to the health challenges in their sub-region. The Arab Maghreb Union: ECCAS and SADC do not have such agencies, while COMESA is trying to set up its own health agency.
- The African CDC and sub-regional health agencies are overdependent on external funding and expertise.

- The absence of a framework within which African countries can develop, promote, and enhance African pharmaceutical production and African traditional medicine. African traditional medicine is despised and marginalised despite the rich knowledge that it embodies.
- It is said that 'he who pays the pipers calls the tune'. Most of Africa's medical research is funded by foreign agencies. In turn, the results belong to the funders.

A new common collective African vision is necessary. It should be negotiated through multilevel governance in a shared sovereignty framework, having its main appeal in the promotion of health cooperation. To this effect, the following suggestions may help to enhance health diplomacy in Africa:

- *Cooperation in funding health research and drug production is imperative.* With the opportunities provided by the World Trade Organisation (WTO) and TRIPS, there is ample room for the African Union to build on the pharmaceutical capacities of selected African countries like Egypt and South Africa to step up the production of cheap generic medicines for the numerous infections plaguing the continent. Investment in health infrastructure is of utmost importance and developing Universal Health Coverage must be incorporated into policies where everyone may have access to health facilities, treatment, and medication.
- *Cooperation in health between and among countries must intensify.* The phenomenon of 'my country first', or 'our sub-region first', must give way to the collective spirit of continental well-being and a collective attainment of health goals.
- *African pharmacopeia and indigenous medicine must be improved and promoted.* The research and development of African pharmacopoeia and indigenous medicine should be incorporated into the health policies and systems of all AU member states. The Africa CDC must consider the need to work with African physiotherapists and traditional practitioners to improve research in those sectors while standardising their practices.
- *An independent evaluation of the state of cooperation in the domain of health is needed.* The African Union should conduct an exhaustive evaluation of the needs and perspectives of health diplomacy and its

ability to help the continent respond to the needs of the African people. Such research should examine the state of preparedness of African countries to face the challenge of auto-financing of health without recourse to external sources.

The 'Africa we want' can only be achieved within the context of robust cooperation among countries of the continent and within the framework of sub-regional groupings working together to make sure African collectivism is achieved to promote African core values in health (Isikalu et al., 2021). Health diplomacy in Africa must be centred on the capacity of regional blocks to take leadership in sustainable health policies and enhance the financial and technical autonomy of the African health system.

REFERENCES

Aidam, J., & Sombie, I. (2016). The West African Health Organization's experience in improving the health research environment in the ECOWAS region. *Health Research Policy and Systems, 14*(30). https://doi.org/10.1186/s12961-016-0102-7

Anderson, E. L. (2018). African health diplomacy: Obscuring power and leveraging dependency through shadow diplomacy. *International Relations. International Relations, 32*(2), 194–217. https://doi.org/10.1177/0047117817751595

AU. (n.d.). *Promoting health and nutrition.* African Union Commission. https://au.int/en/promoting-health-nutrition

AU/Africa CDC. (2022). Africa CDC strengthens the capacity and capability of Africa's public health institutions as well as partnerships to detect and respond quickly and effectively to disease threats and outbreaks, based on data-driven interventions and programmes. https://africacdc.org/.

AUC. (2015, April 1). Africa Regional Nutrition Strategy 2015–2025. African Union. https://au.int/en/documents/20220401/africa-regional-nutrition-strategy-2015-2025.

Brown, G., & Sisskund, D. (2020). International cooperation during the Covid-19 Pandemic. *Oxford Review of Economic Policy, 36*(1), 64–76. https://doi.org/10.1093/oxrep/graa025

Chattu, V. K., Dave, V. B., Reddy, K. S., Singh, B., Sahiledengle, B., Heyi, D. Z., Nattey, C., Atlaw, D., Jackson, K., El-Khatib, Z., & Eltom, A. A. (2021). Advancing African medicines agency through global health diplomacy for an equitable pan-African universal health coverage: A scoping review. *International Journal of Environmental Research and Public Health, 18*(22), 11758. https://doi.org/10.3390/ijerph182211758

COMESA (2016). COMESA Health Framework. https://eproofing.springer. com/ePb/books/dmuZi0ev4zJulSOeHW6h2cGftTHq-fWWLen-miOAPdW- w2mDaDsP0OX1G4mIJ3qkTidEhmQbmk9efBgRDBVvWDeJ18sS1zZBc-oN YSVQRYIEXRor7AEdB2zNP4a-9t72rWUL-bwcovWwvwf0-tpC4Bg==

COMESA. (2022) Ministers endorse procedures to establish COMESA health desk. https://www.comesa.int/.

Department of Social Affairs. (2015). Africa health strategy 2016–2030. *African Union Commission*. https://au.int/sites/default/files/documents/30357- doc-final_ahs_strategy_formatted.pdf.

EA Health. (2022). About EAHRC. https://www.eahealth.org/about-eahrc.

EAC (2018). Health sector investment priority framework 2018–2028. *EAC Secretariat*. https://health.eac.int/publications/eac-health-sector-investment- priority-framework-2018-2028#gsc.tab=0.

EAC. (2022). Health. https://www.eac.int/health.

Fernando, J. (2022). Corporate Social Responsibility (CSR): Explained with Examples. *Investopedia*. www.investopedia.com.

Gupta, A.H.(2021, June 5). How global cooperation could be key to containing the Coronavirus. *The New York Times*. https://www.nytimes. com/2020/06/05/us/coronavirus-who-samantha-power-un.html.

Herpolsheimer, J. (2022, January 11). ECOWAS and the Covid-19 pandemic: Regional responses and African inter-regional cooperation. WATHI. https:// www.wathi.org/ecowas-and-the-covid-19-pandemic-regional-responses- and-african-inter-regional-cooperation/.

Howard-Jones, N. (1975). The scientific background of the international sanitary conferences 1851–1938. *World Health Organization*.. https://apps.who.int/ iris/handle/10665/62873

Isikalu, A. A., Ogu, M. I., & Doma, J. A. (2021). ECOWAS and Strategic Autonomy of the Global South in International Development. *International Journal of Social Sciences and Humanities Reviews, 11*(1), 31–39.

Kaner, J., & Schaack, S. (2016). Understanding Ebola: The 2014 epidemic. *Globalization and Health, 12*, 53. https://doi.org/10.1186/s12992- 016-0194-4

Kelly, L. (2021). Characteristics of global health diplomacy. Knowledge, Evidence, and Learning for Development (K4D). https://opendocs.ids.ac.uk/open- docs/bitstream/handle/20.500.12413/16733/1021_Health_Diplomacy.pdf ?sequence=3&isAllowed=y.

Larbi, H. & Lars, C. (2017). Smart development strategy for the Maghreb: Structural reform, a new role for the state, regional integration. https://www. kas.de/c/document_library/get_file?uuid=3676dc02-4110-6654-8539-cba3 54836aeb&groupId=252038.

Munos, M.M., & Zaid, F.(2022, July 06). The Ministry of Health in Cooperation with UNICEF and WHO, Releases the Assessment Results of WASH and

Infection Prevention Control Services in Health Facilities in Iraq. *UNICEF.* https://www.unicef.org/iraq/press-releases/ministry-health-cooperation-unicef-and-who-releases-assessment-results-wash-and#:~:text=Baghdad%2C%206%20July%202022%E2%80%94%20The,facilities%20in%20Iraq%2C%20with%20the.

Ngandu, K. Y.(2021, April 14). Actions taken by the economic Community of Central African States in response to COVID-19. ACCORD. https://www.accord.org.za/analysis/actions-taken-by-the-economic-community-of-central-african-states-in-response-to-covid-19/.

Penfold, E. D., & Fourie, P. (2015). Regional health governance: A suggested agenda for Southern African Health Diplomacy. *Global Social Policy, 15*(3), 278–795. https://doi.org/10.1177/2F1468018115599817

Pheage, T. (2017, March 17). Dying from lack of medicine: Encouraging local production, rights policies—The way out. *Africa Renewal.* https://www.un.org/africarenewal/magazine/december-2016-march-2017/dying-lack-medicines.

Sahel and West Africa Club Secretariat and OECD. (2014). Ebola does not stop at the border! https://www.oecd.org/swac/ebola.htm.

Southern African Development Community. (n.d.). Health and nutrition. https://www.sadc.int/pillars/health-and-nutrition#:~:text=Strategic%20Development%20Plan-,Health%20Policy%20Framework,to%20high-impact%20health%20interventions

The Africa CDC. (2018). The Africa centres for disease control and prevention emergency operation center support to the government of democratic republic of Congo in *The fight against the ongoing Ebola virus outbreak* in Bikoro. https://africacdc.org/news-item/the-africa-centres-for-disease-control-and-prevention-emergency-operationcenter-support-to-the-government-of-democratic-republic-of-congo-in-the-fight-against-the-ongoing-ebola-virus-outbreak-in-biko/.

UNECA (2016): AMU—Arab Maghreb Union https://archive.uneca.org/

UNECA. (n.d.) The official East African comprehensive compendium of health information. https://www.eahealth.org/.

UNICEF.(2019, July 29). Ebola preparedness and response focus countries: Uganda, South Sudan, Rwanda & Burundi. https://www.unicef.org/esa/ebola-preparedness-and-response.

UNICEF. (2022). World immunisation week 2022: For every child a vaccine. https://www.unicef.org/wca/world-immunization-week-2022.

Valenza, D. (2020, March 30). *The irresistible rise of health diplomacy: Why narratives matter in the time of Covid-19.* United Nations University. https://cris.unu.edu/health-diplomacy-narratives.

WAHO. (2019). 2019 Health situation in the ECOWAS region. West African Health Organisation. https://www.wahooas.org/web-ooas/sites/default/files/publications/2312/health-situation-wa-englishnov2020.pdf.

WHO. (2015). *2015 WHO strategic response plan: West Africa Ebola outbreak.* WHO. https://apps.who.int/iris/bitstream/handle/10665/163360/9789241508698_eng.pdf;jsessionid=249051147FF47E1365D46423E41E FE19?sequence=1

WHO. (2019). SIDS pooled procurement initiative to improve access to quality medicines. WHO: https://www.afro.who.int/news/sids-pooled-procurement-initiative-improve-access-quality-medicines.

WHO (2020, March 10). South African development community unites to tackle COVID-19. World Health Organisation. https://www.afro.who.int/news/south-african-development-community-unites-tackle-covid-19.

CHAPTER 5

Diseases, Epidemics, and Diplomacy in Africa

*Humphrey Ngala Ndi, Henry Ngenyam Bang,
and Emmanuel Etamo Kengo*

INTRODUCTION

Problems of resource governance that have culminated in rampant poverty, conflict, malnutrition in infants, and precarious health systems have connived to give Africa the grimmest medical outlook of all the continental regions of the world. Diseases like malaria, AIDS, and cholera among many others kill more people in Africa than anywhere else. The continent accounts for 95 percent of global malaria cases and 96 percent of malaria deaths

H. N. Ndi (✉)
High Commission for the Republic of Cameroon in London, London, UK

University of Yaounde I, Yaounde, Cameroon

H. N. Bang
Department of Disaster and Emergency Management,
Coventry University, Coventry, UK
e-mail: henry.bang@coventry.ac.uk

E. E. Kengo
Department of History and African Civilizations, University of Buea,
Buea, Cameroon

H. N. Ndi et al. (eds.), *Health Diplomacy in Africa*, Studies in
Diplomacy and International Relations,
https://doi.org/10.1007/978-3-031-41249-3_5

85

(WHO, 2022). Similarly, two-thirds of the 38.4 million people living with HIV/AIDS are found in Africa (WHO, [Nov] 2022). The case of cholera is not different. Cholera originated in the Indian sub-continent and although it is still rampant in Asia, by far the highest mortality from the ailment is recorded in Africa.

Many other infectious diseases with epidemic and pandemic capabilities pose threats to African populations daily. Others like the Ebola virus disease (EVD), almost endemic in the Congo basin, COVID-19, and meningococcal meningitis in Sahelian countries also pose significant health threats to African populations. Their incidence and intensities vary from country to country and are dictated by the adequacy of their health protection and control measures determined by the strengths of their health systems.

Acutely aware of the disease burden of the continent, the African Union has designed numerous policies and strategies aimed at fostering intra-African cooperation and partnerships to fight disease and protect the health of the population at the highest levels of decision-making on the continent. The AIDS WATCH Africa (AWA), a statutory organ of the AU, with representation at the level of heads of state and governments, is set up for advocacy, accountability, and resource mobilisation to build a strong African response to HIV/AIDS, malaria, and tuberculosis. The organ has established useful links with all key organs of the AU such as regional economic groupings, regional health organisations, as well as civil society, the private sector, and agencies that all participate in AU coordination forums. It is therefore a useful platform for health diplomacy among African countries and international organisations. Others are the newly created Africa Centre for Disease Control (CDC), Africa Medicine Agency (AMA), and even the Specialised Technical Committees.

A SNAPSHOT OF PANDEMICS IN AFRICA

The African landmass is extensive and diverse as are its landscapes, peoples, cultures, and economies. By virtue of this diversity, different health challenges affect different parts of the continent at different intensities. From north to south of Africa, one passes through biomes which serve as *geogens* for specific categories of diseases. Those are the cases of meningitis and malaria belts. The origin of the Ebola virus disease (EVD) is traced to the Congo where the virus was first described in 1976, but since 1979, the frequency of outbreaks in the region has increased. Mortality from EVD is situated above 50 percent in most cases. Consequently, as the pace of cross-border travel gathers steam, an outbreak anywhere is a threat to people everywhere on the continent. This is a similar scenario to the more familiar cholera. Above all, despite the occasional threat from EVD and cholera, malaria remains the greatest cause of sickness and death, especially among infants in Africa.

- Malaria

Malaria is a common disease in Sub-Saharan Africa where its transmission is most intense. However, it records very high fatalities in infants. The continent alone accounts for 95 percent of the global cases of the disease. In 2020, an estimated 627 000 Africans died from malaria (WHO, 2022). Though it is endemic in the tropical world where it is spread by the female anopheles mosquito, its effects are less devastating in Asia and the Americas probably due to better prevention, the elimination of mosquitoes, and treatment. Table 5.1 shows the conspicuous position of Africa in the global picture of malaria. However, transmission is not uniform on the continent as the anopheles mosquito does not breed at high altitudes, during cold seasons in some areas, and in deserts excluding oasis. That is why transmission is almost non-existent in the Maghreb and less in the eastern to southern parts of Africa relative to the west and central parts of the continent.

In the areas of highest and year-round transmission, nearly everyone gets a bout of malaria in a year. It is generally underestimated, and most adults do not seek hospital treatment for it. Despite the underestimation,

Table 5.1 Africa and the global situation of malaria, HIV/AIDS, and cholera in 2020

Region	Malaria (%)	HIV/AIDS (%)	Cholera (%)
Africa	95.0	67.0	24
South-East Asia	2.0	10.0	75
Eastern Mediterranean	2.4	1.0	0
Americas	0.3	10	1
Western Pacific	0.7	5.0	0
Europe	0.0	7.0	0

Source: WHO, 2021. (World malaria report 2021); WHO (n.d.). Global HIV programme (https://www.who.int/teams/global-hiv-hepatitis-and-stis-programmes) and WHO (n.d.). Cholera dashboards (https://www.who.int/activities/supporting-cholera-outbreak-response/interactive-summary-visuals-of-cholera-data-officially-reported-to-who-since-2000)

malaria is a severe drain on Africa's economy in terms of lost manhours and the cost of preventing and treating the disease, especially in children to both individuals and the government.

After malaria, an acquired immunodeficiency syndrome (AIDS) is the biggest humanitarian disaster in living memory in Africa. With over 67 percent of all AIDS patients in the world, the continent is the locus of infectives for the disease. Swaziland, Botswana, Lesotho, Malawi, Namibia, Nigeria, Kenya, and Zimbabwe are the most affected. In 2018, over 470,000 people died of AIDS-related illnesses in Africa (WHO, n.d.). The World Health Organisation (WHO) Africa region indicates that AIDS-related deaths have reduced by 45 percent since the first antiretroviral treatment was introduced in the late 1990s. Between 2000 and 2018, thanks to the efforts of national control programmes, civil society advocacy organisations, and international funding, new HIV infections fell by 37 percent. Despite this progress, western and central Africa lag significantly behind eastern and southern Africa in terms of HIV treatment and viral suppression in people living with the virus (UNAIDS, 2017). Overcoming HIV/AIDS in Africa is still a herculean task as the continent still records over 65 percent of all new HIV infections in the world. The challenge of COVID-19 and the sporadic risks of lethal viral infections like the Ebola virus disease (EVD), avian influenza, and many others have diverted significant attention and resources from HIV/AIDS prevention and control, and there are strong signs of its relapse in many African countries.

Outside of malaria, cholera, EVD, and AIDS as diseases with the highest case fatalities in Africa are many other potentially devastating ones. These are described in Table 5.2. A common thread with many of them is their association with the Congo Basin where many zoonotic diseases originate. Humankind's quest for natural resources food and animal products (from wild animals notably apes) has led him to encounter ecosystems that harbour thousands of animal and bird species acting as disease vectors. It is no doubt, therefore, that the Congo Basin is a major fountain of zoonotic infections in Africa.

Disease control and prevention in Africa is important for its role not only in reducing mortality but also in labour protection. In a continent where economic activity is mainly labour intensive, the health of the population is a crucial factor in economic production. A study on the effect of malaria on productivity in a banana plantation in Zimbabwe revealed that most unskilled labourers were absent from work for between 1.5 and 4.1

Table 5.2 Main infectious diseases in Africa

Disease	Prevalence	Fatality rate (percent)
Anthrax	Anthrax is a serious infectious disease caused by gram-positive, rod-shaped bacteria known as *Bacillus anthracis*. Anthrax can be found naturally in soil and commonly affects domestic and wild animals around the world. The disease still exists in animals and humans in most countries of sub-Saharan Africa and Asia, in several southern European countries, in the Americas, and in certain areas of Australia.	20 percent for cutaneous anthrax without antibiotics and 25–75 percent for gastrointestinal anthrax; inhalation anthrax has a fatality rate that is 80 percent or higher
Avian influenza	Avian influenza refers to the disease caused by infection with avian (bird) influenza (flu) Type A viruses. Three subtypes of avian influenza A viruses are known to infect people (H5, H7, and H9 viruses). Among these, Asian lineage H5N1 and H7N9 have caused the majority of infections in people. Extensive outbreaks in poultry have occurred in parts of Africa, Asia, Europe, and the Middle East since 1997, but only sporadic human infections have occurred to date.	Varies from one country to another but generally about 50 percent
Cholera	Cholera is an acute diarrhoeal infection that can kill within hours if left untreated. Caused by the bacterium *Vibrio cholera*. In the past 15 years, over 18 African countries have experienced cholera outbreaks.	With early and proper treatment, the case fatality rate should remain below 1 percent.
COVID-19	COVID-19 is a communicable respiratory infection first reported in China but now spread throughout the world.	About 2 percent (Mahase, E. 2020)

(*continued*)

Table 5.2   (continued)

Disease	Prevalence	Fatality rate (percent)
Crimean-Congo haemorrhagic fever (CCHF)	The Crimean-Congo haemorrhagic fever (CCHF) virus causes severe viral haemorrhagic fever outbreaks. CCHF is endemic in Africa and has a case fatality rate of 40 percent. The virus is primarily transmitted to people from ticks and livestock animals. The disease was first identified in Crimea, but the virus was first isolated in 1956 in the Congo.	40 percent (Africacdc. org)
Dengue	Dengue is a mosquito-borne viral infection. The infection causes flu-like illness and occasionally develops into a potentially lethal complication called severe dengue. Dengue is endemic in tropical and sub-tropical climates	Less than 1 percent if treatment starts early
Ebola virus disease (EVD)	The virus was first discovered in 1976 in the Ebola River region of Congo. Originally transmitted to humans from wild animals (such as fruit bats, porcupines, and non-human primates) and then transmitted from human to human through direct contact with the blood, secretions, organs, or other bodily fluids of an infected person. Outbreaks are recurrent in the Congo Basin countries.	Ebola case fatality rates have varied from 25 percent to 90 percent in past outbreaks. However, with the currently available effective treatment, patients have a significantly higher chance of survival if they are treated early and given supportive care.
Human immunodeficiency syndrome	The human immunodeficiency virus (HIV) is a major global public health challenge that does not have a cure till now. Globally, thirty-five million lives have been affected by this virus. The WHO African region is the most affected region with 25.7 million people living with HIV in 2017. The African region also accounts for over two-thirds of the global total of new HIV infections. The earliest known case of HIV-1 is from the sample taken in 1959 from a man who died in Kinshasa, the Belgian Congo.	4.7 percent

(continued)

Table 5.2   (continued)

Disease	Prevalence	Fatality rate (percent)
Lassa fever	Lassa fever is an acute viral haemorrhagic illness that is endemic in some countries of West Africa. For example, Benin, Ghana, Guinea, Liberia, Mali, Sierra Leone, and Nigeria. The overall case-fatality rate of Lassa fever is 1 percent. The number of Lassa virus infections per year in West Africa is estimated at 100,000 to 300,000, with approximately 5,000 deaths.	1 percent
Malaria	Malaria is transmitted to humans through infected mosquito bites. Although malaria is preventable and curable, it can be a life-threatening condition. In 2016, there were an estimated 216 million cases of malaria in 91 countries with 445,00 deaths, an increase of 5 million cases over 2015 with an approximately similar number of deaths (446,000). In 2016, the WHO AFRO Region represented 90 percent of malaria cases and 91 percent of malaria deaths	A case fatality rate of between 0.01 percent and 0.40 percent was applied to the estimated number of *P. falciparum* cases, and a case fatality rate of between 0.01 percent and 0.06 percent was applied to the estimated number of *P. vivax* cases
Marburg virus disease	Marburg virus disease (MVD), formerly known as Marburg haemorrhagic fever, is a severe, often fatal illness in humans. The Marburg virus is transmitted to people from fruit bats and spreads among humans through human-to-human transmission. It causes severe viral haemorrhagic fever in humans. Outbreaks and sporadic cases have been reported in Angola, the Democratic Republic of Congo, Kenya, and South Africa (in a person with a recent travel history to Zimbabwe).	The case-fatality rate for Marburg haemorrhagic fever is between 23 and to 90 percent.

(*continued*)

Table 5.2 (continued)

Disease	Prevalence	Fatality rate (percent)
Meningococcal meningitis	Meningococcal meningitis is a bacterial form of meningitis, a serious infection of the thin lining that surrounds the brain and spinal cord. Meningococcal meningitis is observed worldwide, but the highest burden of the disease is in the meningitis belt of sub-Saharan Africa, stretching from Senegal in the west to Ethiopia in the east. Around 30 000 cases are still reported each year from that area.	Meningococcal meningitis is associated with high fatality (up to 50 percent when untreated).
Monkeypox	Monkeypox is a rare, viral zoonotic disease that is caused by the monkeypox virus. It occurs primarily in tropical rainforest areas of central and west Africa. Monkeypox can spread in humans through close contact, often skin-to-skin contact, with an infected person or animal, or with material contaminated with the virus such as clothing, bedding, and towels. It was first identified in humans in the Democratic Republic of the Congo in 1970.	3–6 percent
Poliomyelitis	Poliomyelitis (polio) is a highly infectious disease caused by a virus. Polio mainly affects children under 5 years of age. Cases due to wild poliovirus have decreased by over 99 percent since 1988, from an estimated 350 000 cases then to 22 reported cases in 2017. As a result of the global effort to eradicate the disease, more than 16 million people have been saved from paralysis.	Generally, 2 percent to 5 percent among children and up to 15 percent to 30 percent among adolescents and adults.

(*continued*)

Table 5.2   (continued)

Disease	Prevalence	Fatality rate (percent)
Yellow fever	Yellow fever is an acute viral haemorrhagic disease transmitted through infected mosquitoes. It was named yellow as it, sometimes, causes jaundice (yellow skin and eyes) in infected people. Thirty-four African countries are endemic to yellow fever. It is thought to have originated in Central or East Africa and spread to Europe and the Americas in the slave trade movements.	The case fatality rate of severe yellow fever is 50 percent or higher

Sources: AU/Africa CDC, n.d.; https://africacdc.org/disease/; USFDA, February 2018; https://www.fda.gov/vaccines-blood-biologics/vaccines/anthrax

days in a five-month survey period (Lukwa et al., 2019). How entrenched the effects of malaria may be on economic productivity depends not only on geography but also on the ability of individual countries to implement suitable and effective control and eradication programmes. Malaria and poverty are thus intimately connected (Gallup & Sachs, 2001). Mauritius Island once severely malarious is a suitable example that illustrates the success of the prevention of malaria transmission that was achieved in 1998 (Tatarsky et al., 2011).

DIPLOMATIC COOPERATION IN EPIDEMICS AND PANDEMICS IN AFRICA

In a world which has become very globalised characterised by fast-paced international movements of people and merchandise notably by air, it has become impossible for a single country acting on its own to protect its citizens from virulent viral and bacterial infections which now occur on an increasing frequency. The pathogenicity of emerging and re-emerging viruses like the Ebola virus disease, bird flu or avian influenza (H5N1), and swine flu (H1N1) among many others poses a permanent risk to human populations worldwide. In response to this risk, the International Health Regulations, an instrument of international law, was negotiated to define the rights and obligations of state parties in responding to cross-border public health emergencies.

The International Health Regulations (IHR) 2005 is an international instrument that is legally binding on all World Health Organisation member states. Their objective is to prevent, protect people against, and control the international spread of disease. Having been ratified by over 196 countries, it is the biggest concerted diplomatic approach to international health protection to date.

The institutional framework for health diplomacy in Africa is generally provided by the African Union which defines one of its objectives as the eradication of preventable diseases and the promotion of good health on the continent through cooperation with relevant internal partners. Although that speaks to the legendary dependence of the continent on international aid, it is also true that such cooperation has resulted in remarkable improvements in the health of millions of Africans.

THE INSTITUTIONAL ARCHITECTURE OF AFRICAN HEALTH DIPLOMACY

The African Union has created an armada of organs to push out the frontiers of health policy formulation and implementation among its members. The supreme decision-making organ of the AU is The Assembly of Heads of States and Government which meets once a year. Among other rules, it determines the common policies of the Union; establishes new organs for the Union; adopts its budget; gives directives to the Executive Council on the management of conflicts, war, and other emergencies; and appoints the Chair and Vice-Chair of the AU Commission and the Commissioners.

Immediately below the Assembly of Heads of State and Government is the Executive Council. It is composed of Ministers of Foreign Affairs of member countries, or any personalities designated by their governments. It meets twice yearly but may also meet in extraordinary sessions at the request of a Member State. The Council coordinates and takes decisions on policies of common interest to member states. Health, disaster relief, and response are a few of the many domains of its competence. The Council is responsible to the Assembly, and it may also delegate any of its powers and functions to the Specialised Technical Committees (STC) of the AU. There is an STC on Health, Labour, and Social Affairs.

The African Union (AU) Commission, acting as a secretariat, runs the routine business of the AU. The Commission is made up of nine departments among which are Health, Humanitarian Affairs and Social Development (HHS). The HHS oversees the policy and strategic development and execution of the decisions of AU policy organs in the areas of Health, Humanitarian Affairs and Social Development. It has two directorates, five divisions, and ten specialised institutions. One of the specialised institutions is the Africa CDC.

The Directorate of Health and Humanitarian Affairs oversees policy implementation in the areas of health and humanitarian affairs such as health issues related to health policy and delivery systems, nutrition and other related public health issues and challenges. It plays a frontline role in policy development, advocacy, coordination, monitoring and evaluation of AIDS, tuberculosis and malaria, and other infectious diseases. It also provides a strategic orientation for addressing humanitarian crises in sustainable ways. The division of health systems, diseases, and nutrition responds to vital generic health issues related to health policy and delivery systems, nutrition and other related public health issues and challenges that require a concerted and coordinated approach at a continental level. The division further plays a leading role in policy development, advocacy, coordination, monitoring and evaluation of AIDS, tuberculosis and malaria, and other infectious diseases.

AWA is a statutory entity of the AU with the specific mandate to lead advocacy, accountability, and resource mobilisation efforts for a robust African response to end AIDS, tuberculosis, and malaria by 2030. It is hosted within the division of Health Systems, Diseases and Nutrition, Directorate of Health, and Humanitarian Affairs. Other AU organs created to improve Africa's institutional response to disease are the Partnership for African Vaccine Manufacturing and the African Medicine Agency.

This chapter uses the case of the fight against the HIV/AIDS pandemic in Africa to illustrate the importance of international cooperation in responding to health emergencies.

AFRICA'S MULTILATERAL PARTNERS AND THE FIGHT AGAINST HIV/AIDS

The UNO has been a crucial partner to Africa in the continent's struggles against the HIV/AIDS pandemic. Perhaps, the greatest global diplomatic effort at responding to the pandemic was the General Assembly Declaration of Commitment to doubling up the fight against the pandemic adopted at its twenty-sixth special session (UNGA, 2001). Concerned by the health and economic devastation caused by HIV which had infected over 36.1 million people at the end of the year 2000, with 75 percent being in sub-Saharan Africa, heads of State and Governments or their representatives pledged to secure a global commitment to enhancing coordination and intensification of national, regional, and international efforts to comprehensively combat HIV/AIDS in all its aspects. The commitment covered ten actions that member countries and international partners had to undertake.

The first of them was leadership. Governments, complemented by the active participation of civil society organisations, and the private sector were encouraged to lead the fight against HIV/AIDS through concrete actions.

- At the national level, public and private sector stakeholders committed to addressing the epidemic by confronting stigma, silence, and denial; addressing the gender- and age-based dimensions of the epidemic; eliminating discrimination and marginalisation; and forging partnerships with civil society, the business community, and pushing for the full participation of people living with HIV/AIDS. Furthermore, governments committed to integrating HIV/AIDS prevention, care, treatment, support, and impact mitigation priorities into development planning programmes, poverty reduction strategies, national budget allocations, and sectoral development plans by 2003.
- At the regional and sub-regional level, governments committed to being actively involved in addressing the HIV/AIDS crisis through cooperation and coordination. They resolved to support regional and sub-regional initiatives such as the International Partnership against AIDS in Africa (IPAA) and the ECA-African Development Forum African Consensus and Plan of Action: Leadership to overcome HIV/AIDS; the Abuja Declaration and the Framework for Action for the fight against HIV/AIDS, tuberculosis, and other related infectious diseases in Africa, among others.

The second component of the declaration was for governments and partners to make prevention the backbone of the response to the pandemic to achieve the internationally agreed global prevention goal to reduce HIV prevalence among young men and women aged 15 to 24 in the most affected countries by 25 percent in 2005 and globally by another 25 percent in 2010.

Other components of the Declaration included care, support, and treatment of HIV/AIDS patients; integration of human rights into the fight against HIV/AIDS through legislation, regulations, and other measures that eliminate all forms of discrimination and stigmatisation of people living with HIV/AIDS; increased investments in research and development to find a possible cure for HIV/AIDS; finding additional and sustained resources for HIV/AIDS; and maintaining the momentum against HIV/AIDS by following up and monitoring all initiatives against the ailment.

Remarkable progress has been made since this declaration was made in 2001. This has been due to the targets set unanimously by over 150 Heads of State and Governments, private sector, and civil society actors to halt HIV/AIDS and ensure that it begins to be reversed by 2015. The UN General Assembly supported the establishment of a Global HIV/AIDS Health Fund for prevention, care, support, and treatment (UNGA, 2006). No doubt, the propulsion for this global awakening came from the decision by several major pharmaceutical companies to drastically cut antiretroviral drug prices for the most affected countries, on the one hand, and heightened commitment from many rich countries to fight the scourge on the other. The 1995 WTO agreement on trade-related aspects of intellectual property rights (TRIPS) and the possibilities it offered pharmaceutical companies to waive some aspects of the agreement to produce generic drugs for public health emergencies was a definite game changer in the struggle against HIV/AIDS in sub-Saharan Africa as it resulted in cheaper drugs and more people gaining access to antiretroviral treatment.

TRIPS Flexibilities and the Negotiation of Generic HIV/AIDS Medicines

Perhaps, the most important component of United Nations General Assembly resolution S-26/2 on the declaration on HIV/AIDS (UNGA, 2001) was the effort to overcome barriers to pricing, tariffs and trade agreements, procurement, and supply chain management to fast-track and intensify access to affordable and good-quality HIV/AIDS prevention and diagnostic products, as well as medicines. If this declaration was to be transformed into reality, the World Trade Organisation had to play a critical role through its agreement on the TRIPS. The agreement requires that pharmaceutical patents should be protected for at least 20 years to enable inventors to recover the cost of their invention and reinvest more resources into research and development activities. As such, the inspiration behind TRIPS is not only the reward of innovation and invention but also the enhancement of further research and inventions. Resolution 60/262 of the UN General Assembly of 2006 reaffirms that TRIPS should not be employed to prevent member countries from taking measures to protect public health. Rather, it should be interpreted in a manner that is supportive of the right to protect public health and improve access to medicine for all, including the production of generic antiretroviral drugs and other essential medicines for AIDS-related infections. This is where deliberate international cooperation and partnerships is crucial. The lobbying efficiency of civil society organisations and non-governmental organisations has also been registered here. Somehow, the Doha Declaration on the TRIPS and Public Health acknowledges the importance of public health and highlights the right of countries to make use of the flexibilities available within the agreement to increase access to medicines for countries with low or no pharmaceutical production capacity. This caveat in the TRIPS agreement has been exploited by countries like India, Brazil, Indonesia, and Thailand to produce cheap generic drugs that have helped reduce the cost of preventing and treating HIV/AIDS in developing countries notably in Africa. This is reflected in the enormous progress registered in the response to the pandemic. Today, over 57 percent of all people living with HIV know their status; 46 percent are accessing treatment; and 38 percent have suppressed viral loads (UNAIDS, 2017). The implication of virally suppressed HIV is that it can no longer be transmitted.

Exploiting the TRIPS flexibilities, the Indian pharmaceutical giant, CIPLA, was the first company to cut down the cost of antiretroviral therapy. The company produced and offered a fixed-dose triple-combination antiretroviral therapy to non-governmental organisations in Africa at US$350 per patient per year and to African governments at US$ 600 per patient per year in 2001 (UNAIDS, 2016). This offers revolutionised HIV treatment in developing countries resulting in the enhanced decline in HIV/AIDS mortality on the African continent. According to the Africa WHO Regional Office, 470,000 people died of HIV/AIDS in 2018. This represented a 40 percent decline from 2010 (WHO, 2021). In November 2015, the WTO TRIPS Council adopted an extension of the TRIPS exemption over pharmaceutical products for the least developed countries until January 2033 (ibid.).

Under circumstances of severe emergency, the agreement allows for the government use of compulsory licensing. In instances of public health emergencies, governments may temporarily license a patented product without the consent of the patent holder. By 2010, 17 low- to middle-income countries had issued temporary licences for government use of anti-retroviral medicines. In addition to temporary licensing, another mechanism for increasing access to pharmaceutical products and health technologies is the use of voluntary licensing agreements, whereby a patent holder allows another party to use the patent rights under defined conditions, often, but not always in exchange for payment of an agreed royalty. Many pharmaceutical companies have used voluntary licensing agreements to extend HIV treatments and the use of life-saving medicines through the Medicines Patent Pool (MPP), an UN-backed initiative.

Africa could have been the greatest beneficiary of TRIPS flexibilities if it had a strong capacity to produce pharmaceuticals. It has 32 of the 44 countries classified as least developed globally. The least developed countries (LDCs) refer to those territories listed by the UN as having or confronting severe structural impediments to sustainable development. Their TRIPS privileges for pharmaceuticals last only up to 2033 when they will be obliged to abide by intellectual property standards under TRIPS.

The Prospects for Health Diplomacy in Africa

The African Union Constitutive Act envisioned that the organisation would work with relevant international partners to eradicate preventable diseases and promote good health on the continent. The health mandate of the organisation is implemented by the African Union Commissioner for Social Affairs through the Division for Health and Humanitarian Affairs and Health Systems Disease and Nutrition Division. Whereas the former addresses issues related to health policy, health care delivery systems, nutrition, and any related health problems that require concerted or coordinated approaches at the continental level; the latter is more involved in health policy advocacy, coordination, monitoring, and evaluation of the progress in the prevention, treatment, and management of key diseases like AIDS, tuberculosis, malaria, and other infectious diseases.

Pursuant to the newly created AU, AWA was created in 2001 at the AU Abuja Summit on HIV/AIDS, TB, and other related infectious diseases.

Eight Heads of State and Government established AWA as the arm of the AU focused on African-led advocacy and accountability to press for the urgent acceleration of action to combat the AIDS epidemic. AWA's mandate was expanded to include malaria and TB during its revitalisation in 2012. During the Millennium Development Goals (MDGs) era, the AWA platform changed the African response to HIV/AIDS, TB, and malaria from traditional biomedical and behavioural approaches and catapulted it to transformative enablers focusing on diversified health financing, access to affordable and quality-assured medicines, leadership, governance, and accountability as the path to universal access to health.

AWA's unique mandate empowers it with a role as a convener, directly leveraging the highest level leadership of the AU Member States into action. Across the globe, there is compelling evidence and proof that top political leadership is paramount to building and sustaining actions to defeat AIDS, TB, and malaria. AWA has a 'seat at the table' and occupies a distinct space in global health. It is recognised as a historic triumph of Africa's visionary leadership in health development and governance. The platform has played an influential advocacy role by increasing resource allocation to health in countries and mobilising global resources including the establishment of global institutions supporting programmes in AIDS, TB, and malaria. These programmes include the Global Fund to Fight AIDS, TB, and malaria, established in 2002, which has had a profound effect on reducing the incidence of these three deadly diseases. AWA's role in working with Heads of State to provide financial resources to the Global Fund continues to help the Fund leverage global contributions during its replenishment cycles.

To further enhance the health promotion and protection role of the AU, specialised technical agencies have been created by the organisation to improve the continent's responses to diseases, epidemics, and pandemics. To that effect, the special technical committee (STC) on *Health, Population and Drug Control* and the *African Centres for Diseases Control and Prevention (Africa CDC)* were created in 2015 and 2017, respectively, to transmute this vision into reality.

The STC is charged with identifying areas of cooperation and establishing mechanisms for regional, continental, and global collaboration. The STCs are composed of Ministers or senior officials responsible for sectors falling within their respective areas of competence. There is an STC on Health, Population, and Drug Control which reviews progress on the implementation of continental policies, strategies, programmes, and decisions in the three sectors of its competence. The committee identifies areas of cooperation and establishes mechanisms for regional, continental, and global cooperation. It further serves to elaborate Common African Positions in its three areas and advises relevant AU policy organs on priority programmes and their impact on improving lives.

On its part, the Africa CDC seeks to strengthen Africa's public health institutional capacities and capabilities to detect and respond quickly and efficiently to disease threats and outbreaks based on scientific evidence and data-driven policies and programmes. Among many other objectives, the agency aims at:

- establishing early warning and response systems that address health threats including infectious and chronic disease and during natural disasters;
- strengthening health security in Africa by helping member states comply with international health regulations (IHR);
- hazard and disease mapping;
- strengthening health systems;
- harmonising disease control and prevention policies and surveillance systems in member states;
- promote partnership and collaboration among member states to address emerging and endemic diseases.

Added to the role of STCs, the high-level meetings of African Ministers of Health also constitute an authentic platform for cooperation in health. In the ongoing COVID-19 pandemic, African Ministers of Health are playing an active role in coordinating the continental approach to the virus. They have committed to supporting the approach initiated by the Africa CDC entailing prevention, monitoring, and treatment of the virus. To boost their bargaining leverage, the Ministers called on the AU Member States to take up their COVID-19 orders through the African Vaccine Acquisition Task Team platform and to liaise with the African Export-Import Bank to arrange for the advance purchases of vaccines.

The Africa CDC has positioned itself as the undisputed torchbearer of health cooperation on the continent. Initiatives like the Partnerships for African Vaccine manufacturing (PAVM) and the Institute of Pathogen Genomics (IPG) have the potential to incite and sustain scientific, technological, and medical policy towards vaccine/pharmaceutical autonomy in Africa.

The Partnerships for African Vaccine Manufacturing (PAVM) was established by the African Union (AU) in 2021 to enable the African vaccine manufacturing industry to develop, produce, and supply over 60 percent of the total vaccine doses required on the continent by 2040, up from less than 1 percent today (with interim goals of 10 percent by 2025 and 30 percent by 2030). African leaders met in April 2021 to map out a path to achieve this ambition and agreed on the need for a strong continental strategy adapted to regional specificities—a Framework for Action (FFA). Since then, the Africa Centres for Disease Control and Prevention has worked with stakeholders across the continent to shape a detailed FFA that lays out the key interventions required to enable the development of a viable vaccine manufacturing industry in Africa. Currently, local African manufacturing supplies approximately 1 percent of the total continental demand and manufacturers are consolidated across just five countries (South Africa, Morocco, Tunisia, Egypt, and Senegal). The rest of the supplies come from global providers, including established suppliers in India who provided 70 percent of Vaccine Alliance supply and up to 40 percent for self-procuring countries. The rest of the supply is accounted for by large multinational pharmaceutical corporations notably Merck, Sanofi, Pfizer, and GSK or large, incumbent developing countries vaccine manufacturers (DCVMs).

The FFA is built on the premise that Africa can and should adopt a fully integrated ecosystem to generate investment in all steps of the vaccine manufacturing and supply chain—including research and development, drug substance, and fill and finish. The FFA recommends greater investment in DS manufacturing for vaccines critical for the continent.

With this integrated ecosystem approach in mind, the FFA prioritises the manufacturing of vaccines for 22 diseases identified as critical. These comprise vaccines for ten legacy diseases (including tuberculosis, hepatitis B, and measles), which are typically high-volume and can offer economies of scale, six expanding diseases that typically do not yet have commoditised vaccines or have relatively higher-priced vaccines (including key pandemic and endemic diseases for which vaccines are needed such as HIV, malaria, and COVID-19); and six outbreak diseases (including Ebola). A focus on these diseases should address the continent's pressing patient needs through vaccines that would be feasible and attractive to manufacture. Some of the prioritised diseases have vaccines that have already been developed, so the need is for local production and access. Other vaccines under development could be brought to fruition and subsequently produced on the continent. To achieve this, African governments must mobilise US$30 billion over the next 20 years (2021–2041).

Added to the Africa CDC is the African Medicines Agency (AMA), created by the treaty in February 2019 at the 32nd Session of the Assembly of Heads of State and Government. It is hoped that AMA will enhance the capacity of States Parties and Regional Economic Communities (RECs) to regulate medical products in order to improve access to quality, safe and efficacious medical products in Africa. It is anticipated that all countries will ratify the treaty to enhance the credibility of the agency. In March 2021, less than 20 of Africa's 54 countries had ratified the AMA treaty (AU, 2021). AMA will be the second continental health agency after the Africa CDC, which will enhance the capacity of States Parties and Regional Economic Communities (RECs) to regulate medical products in order to improve access to quality, safe, and efficacious medical products on the continent. It is also hoped that AMA will promote the adoption and harmonisation of medical products regulatory policies and standards, as well as provide scientific guidelines and coordinate existing regulatory harmonisation efforts by the African Union and the regional economic communities (RECs).

At the AU commission level, there is a strong desire to coordinate the efforts of Member States, African Union Agencies, the World Health Organisation, and other partners to ensure synergy and minimise duplication. Added to this, the eight recognised regional groupings of the African Union offer great scope for health diplomacy in their spheres. Most of them have an important health protection and promotion component. This is indicative of the importance of health in the political, economic, and security agenda of the organisations. Table 5.3 presents the health structures of the regional groupings and their objectives.

The Community Health Workers initiative

The HIV/AIDS scourge remains a critical barrier to social and economic development in Africa. In 2017, cognisant of this, African Heads of State endorsed two major initiatives to help end AIDS by 2030. These are the Community Health Workers initiative which aims to recruit, train and deploy two million community health workers across Africa by 2020, and the western and central Africa catch-up Plan to step up access to HIV treatment in these regions which lag behind the eastern and southern African regions in HIV/AIDS prevention and management. The

Table 5.3   Regional groupings of the African Union

African Union/ Regional Groups	Members	Health promotion and protection structure	Objective
The African Union	53 African countries	AU Commission for Social Affairs (Divisions for Health, Nutrition and Population; HIV/AIDS; malaria; tuberculosis; and other infectious diseases	To respond to vital generic health issues related to health policy and delivery systems, nutrition and related public health issues and challenges that require a concerted, and coordinated approach at a continental level. Plays a leading advocacy, monitoring and evaluation role on AIDS, tuberculosis, malaria, and other infectious diseases.
The Arab Maghreb Union (AMU)	Algeria, Libya, Mauritania, Morocco, Tunisia	–	–
The Economic Community of West African States (ECOWAS)	Benin, Burkina Faso, Cabo Verde, Cote d'Ivoire, Gambia, Ghana, Guinea, Guinea Bissau, Liberia, Mali, Niger, Nigeria, Senegal, Sierra Leone, and Togo	The West African Health Organisation	The West African Health Organisation works for the attainment of the highest possible standard and protection of the health of the people in the sub-region through the harmonisation of the policies of the Member States, pooling of resources, and cooperation with one another and with others for collective and strategic combat against the health problems of the sub-region'.

(*continued*)

Table 5.3 (continued)

African Union/ Regional Groups	Members	Health promotion and protection structure	Objective
The East African Community (EAC)	Democratic Republic of the Congo, Tanzania, Kenya, Burundi, Rwanda, South Sudan, and Uganda	East African Community Health Department	Undertakes joint action towards the prevention and control of communicable and non-communicable diseases and controls pandemics and epidemics of communicable and vector-borne diseases that might endanger the health and welfare of the residents of the community. Cooperates in facilitating mass immunisation and other public health community campaigns.
The Intergovernmental Authority on Development (IGAD)	Djibouti, Eritrea, Ethiopia, Kenya, Somalia, South Sudan, Sudan, Uganda	Division of Health and Social Development	–

(*continued*)

Table 5.3 (continued)

African Union/ Regional Groups	Members	Health promotion and protection structure	Objective
South African Development Community (SADC)	Angola, Botswana, Comoros, Democratic Republic of the Congo, Eswatini, Lesotho, Madagascar, Malawi, Mauritius, Mozambique, Namibia, Seychelles, South Africa, Tanzania, Zambia, and Zimbabwe	The Social and Human Development and Special Programmes Directorate runs three programmes: the health policy framework; the SADC Protocol on Health; and the Regional Indicative Strategic Development Plan	Recognising that a healthy population is a necessary catalyst for economic and social development, SADC considers the health of its citizens paramount in ensuring a sustainable future. The Southern African Development Community (SADC) is committed to the health of the region's citizens. It aims to attain an acceptable standard of health for all citizens and to reach specific targets within the objective of 'Health for All' by 2020.

(*continued*)

Table 5.3 (continued)

African Union/ Regional Groups	Members	Health promotion and protection structure	Objective
The Common Market for Eastern and Southern Africa (COMESA)	Burundi, Comoros, Democratic Republic of the Congo, Djibouti, Egypt, Eritrea, Eswatini, Ethiopia, Kenya, Libya, Madagascar, Mauritius, Rwanda, Seychelles, Somalia, Sudan, Tunisia, and Uganda	COMESA Health Framework	The COMESA Health Framework seeks to ensure that the region is free from the threat of preventable communicable and non-communicable diseases and death in tandem with the Abuja +12 2030, Target Catalytic Framework to End HIV/AIDS, TB, and malaria by 2030, the Ending the AIDS Epidemic 90-90-90 Strategy, and the UN Sustainable Development Goal No. 3. Specifically, the framework is meant to strengthen national and regional health systems and infrastructure;
The Economic Community of Central African States (ECCAS)	Angola, Burundi, Cameroon, Central African Republic, Chad, Congo, Democratic Republic of the Congo, Equatorial Guinea, Gabon, Rwanda, Sao Tome, and Principe.	Division of Health and Social Affairs	The control of tuberculosis, trypanosomiasis, leprosy, treponematosis, bilharzia, measles, cerebrospinal meningitis, malaria, onchocerciasis, intestinal parasitosis, vaccinations, health education and Reduces the prevalence in Central Africa of communicable diseases.

(*continued*)

Table 5.3 (continued)

African Union/ Regional Groups	Members	Health promotion and protection structure	Objective
The Community of Sahel-Sahara States (CENSAD)	Benin, Burkina Faso, Central African Republic, Comoros, Cote d'Ivoire, Djibouti, Eritrea, Gambia, Ghana, Guinea Bissau, Libya, Mali, Mauritania, Morocco, Niger, Nigeria, Senegal, Sierra Leone, Somalia, Sudan, Togo, and Tunisia	–	–
The Economic and Monetary Community of Central Africa (CEMAC)	Cameroon, Central African Republic, Chad, Equatorial Guinea, Gabon, and Congo	Organisation for coordinating the fight against endemics in central Africa	The actions of OCEAC were oriented towards the fight against tuberculosis, trypanosomiasis, leprosy, treponematosis, schistosomiasis, measles, cerebrospinal meningitis, malaria, onchocerciasis, intestinal parasites, vaccinations, health education, among others.

percentage of people living with HIV who know their status in western and central Africa is barely 36 percent, compared with 62 percent in eastern to southern Africa; those who are on antiretroviral therapy is 28 percent in western and central Africa, compared to 54 percent in eastern to southern Africa; and those with a virally suppressed HIV status are 12 percent and 45 percent, respectively. In order to achieve the 90-90-90 target by December 2020, the region's HIV strategy had to be fast-tracked. This initiative hopes that by 2020, 90 percent of all those living with HIV will know their status; 90 percent of all those diagnosed with the virus will be receiving antiretroviral therapy; and 90 percent of all those on treatment will have viral suppression (UNAIDS, 2014).

The two million Community Health Workers initiative is a direct response to the 90-90-90 targets. It is hoped that the recruitment of 2 million community health workers will be crucial in achieving such socio-economic transformation in Africa that reduces or eliminates the stigma around HIV/AIDS, encouraging more people to seek voluntary testing and antiretroviral treatments. The Joint United Nations Programme on HIV/AIDS (UNAIDS) estimates that there are one million community health workers in Africa. Although they are influential in their communities, most focus on a single health problem, are undertrained, unpaid or underpaid and not well integrated into the health system. Building on this observation, the new initiative shall aim at retraining existing Community Health Workers where feasible and recruiting new health workers to reach the 2 million target.

THE WESTERN AND CENTRAL AFRICA CATCH-UP PLAN

The plan aims at radically accelerating HIV testing, prevention, and treatment in the western and central African region as a levelling up measure with eastern and southern Africa. At least 10 countries (Benin, Cameroon, the Central African Republic, Côte d'Ivoire, the Democratic Republic of the Congo, Guinea, Liberia, Nigeria, Senegal, and Sierra Leone) are already implementing country operational plans deriving from the western and central Africa catch-up plan and tangible progress is witnessed in terms of the desired policy changes and structural changes, but the speed is yet to be optimal, and the new trajectory is yet to be attained.

The first phase started in late 2016 and was focused on eight countries with significant shares of people newly infected with HIV and with treatment coverage of less than 36 percent. These are Cameroon, Côte d'Ivoire, the Democratic Republic of the Congo and Nigeria, and countries with weak health systems that were exposed during the Ebola outbreak and have an urgent need to fast-track their HIV response. These were Guinea, Liberia, Sierra Leone, and the Central African Republic.

The second phase has already started and is gradually extending to the rest of the countries. The main activities are country consultations, identification of barriers and solutions, cross learning with countries already implementing the plan, and the development of respective country plans. In this group, a growing number of countries have already expressed a renewed political commitment to speed up the HIV response in the wake of the catch-up plan and are developing and implementing catch-up plans, in Benin, Burkina Faso, Chad, Equatorial Guinea, Gabon, and Senegal. These country plans address the following crucial success factors:

- Country ownership and political leadership.
- Reconfigured service delivery: task shifting and community service delivery.
- Uninterrupted supplies of commodities: test kits, antiretroviral medicines, early infant diagnosis, as well as viral load kits.

The latest test of the AU's commitment to a continent-wide response to a pandemic was its initiatives against COVID-19. Thanks to its institutional reforms in public health that culminated in the formation of the Africa CDC, the AU was able to respond in a proactive manner to the virus. Through the Partnership to Accelerate COVID-19 Testing (PACT), the Africa CDC worked to trace, test, and track the pandemic across the continent. PACT concentrates on warehousing or product storage and the establishment of distribution hubs across Africa, in conjunction with the World Food Programme and Ethiopian Airlines (Alden & Dunst, 2020). With this capability, the partnership hoped that 10 million Africans would be tested in the six months that followed the start of the pandemic.

In spite of the AU's impressive health diplomacy institutions, the continent's dizzying financial problems compounded by heavy indebtedness compel the AU as well as individual countries to look out of the continent for help to fight pandemics. In the immediate aftermath of the COVID-19 pandemic, Moussa Faki Mahamat, the Chairman of the African Union Commission declared emphatically that the African continent needed finances to deal with the COVID-19 crisis from a health point of view and to deal with all the humanitarian needs that would appear in future (AUC, 2015). While external resources are important in addressing health crises and disasters, they do not enable the development of robust health systems with integrated mechanisms for fighting emergencies on the continent.

The Challenges of Health Diplomacy in Africa

The emergence of new infectious diseases and the increasing frequency of viral infections today make health cooperation an indispensable component of multilateral as well as bilateral diplomacy. The COVID-19 pandemic is a case in point. It has shown that fighting a pandemic in a disconcerted manner yields little results because the existence of the virus anywhere is a risk to people everywhere. The current global diplomatic push for richer countries to share some of their COVID-19 vaccine stocks with the poorer ones led by the Global Vaccine Alliance within the COVID-19 Vaccines Global Access (COVAX) is an illustration of the persistence of health considerations in diplomacy and foreign policy considerations. The UN General Assembly Resolution 63/33 not only recognises the close relationship between foreign policy and global health and their interdependence but also urges states to consider health issues in the formulation of foreign policy because global challenges require concerted and sustained action by the international community (UNGA, 2009). According to Resolution 63/33, a note by the UN Secretary-General to the 64th Session of the General Assembly identified key challenges confronting foreign policymakers.

- *Over-reliance on external resources*

By far the greatest challenge to health cooperation in Africa is the continent's over-reliance on external funding for its social and economic development programmes. Beginning from the African Union (AU), a pan-African project which is almost entirely funded by international partners and not member countries, the dire image of intra-African cooperation in health is laid bare. The AU is funded by contributions from its 55 member states and by donations from external partners. In 2005, AU member states decided that Algeria, Egypt, Libya, Nigeria, and South Africa, the five biggest economies on the continent would contribute 75 percent of the organisation's finances (Pharatlhatlhe & Vanheukelom, 2019). Although the remaining 50 countries had to contribute only 25 percent, by 2015, the AU was able to collect only 67 percent of this proportion on average, with over 30 member states fully or partially defaulting on their payments each year (ibid.). The advent of the Arab Spring dealt a devastating blow to the AU finances because Libya dropped from among the five major donors and Algeria was significantly shaken.

Furthermore, few African countries enjoy sustained economic growth rates and are often caught in internal and regional conflicts that exacerbate problems related to food sufficiency, health care, and infrastructural development. As such only a few states are consistently able to pay their annual financial contributions to the organisation. In the face of its precarious financial standing, the AU has embraced external funding. Surprisingly, external funding is not a negligible complementary appendix to the organisation's budget, but rather the main source of its programme budget. Out of a budget of US$ 647,379,441 in 2019, over US$401,439,576, representing 56.75 percent, was expected to come from international donors (AU, 2020). In this scenario, there is a strong temptation to think that the AU budget may reflect donor rather than African priorities. For example, 70 percent of donor funding is directed to peacekeeping activities as a priority, rather than the programme budget. This is frequently driven by the desire to safeguard the political and economic interests of the ruling elites and key international actors (Pharatlhatlhe & Vanheukelom, 2019). Assessing the chances of success for the African pharmaceutical sector, Dr Margaret Agama-Anyetei, Head of the Division for Health, Nutrition and Population at the AU, underscores the challenges of inadequate and unsustainable funding mechanisms for achieving the continent's pharmaceutical initiatives (African Union, n.d.).

Donor dependency for health programmes is also replicated at individual country levels. Country budgets are also drawn up with significant allowance reserved for international aid. Few health programmes in SSA are funded entirely by state budgets. Ndi (2021) notes that May 2020, the IMF Executive Board approved a US$226 million loan to Cameroon to address the economic impact of the COVID-19 pandemic. The WHO, World Bank, UNICEF, *Médecins Sans frontieres*, UNISAID, the Bill and Melinda Foundation, and many others support or fund health programmes in individual African countries. Health care and disease control programmes in many of these countries would not fully run without external funding. In Cameroon, the Ministry of Public Health has benefitted from the generous aid of the USA to fight epidemic disease like malaria and AIDS (PEPFAR, 2020). Other partners in this programme are Plan International and the Centres for Disease Control and Prevention. Similarly, Cameroon's national antimalaria committee benefitted over US$32.9 million from international donors, compared with US$6.5 million from the government of the country (PMI, 2022). Africa's overdependence on external assistance for social development is the result of its low global economic profile whose origins date back to the transatlantic slave trade, followed by European colonialism and imperialism that instituted a world economic system that maintains Africa as a producer and trader in raw materials keeping her in a subjugated and economically uncompetitive situation that has continued to favour the economic exploitation of the continent (Hickel, 2017). In the post-independence period, this has been compounded by nepotistic and corrupt political leadership that has promoted self-destructive policies for so long that the continent's development has slipped so far behind that of its peers in Asia and South America. Weak economic production has resulted in low investments in education, research, and knowledge production. Only 0.4 percent of the GDP in SSA goes for scientific research, and research and development compared to 27 percent, 31 percent, and 37 percent for Europe, Asia, and North America, respectively (Olufadewa et al., 2020). Fonn (2018) notes that in 2008, Africa produced 27000 scientific publications, the same number as the Netherlands, putting the continent's global scientific output at less than 1 percent. With such a low level of research funding, it is very unlikely that individual African countries can be able to deal with their deplorable states of health without external assistance.

- *Africa's shared loyalties and the plight of health cooperation*

Related to over-dependence is Africa's shared loyalties between itself and its donor partners. Africa's reliance on foreign aid is chronic and the continent seems to have entered a vicious cycle of borrowing with no end in sight. Although overseas development assistance (ODA) is often framed as the desire of the donor to promote development and combat poverty, subtle public diplomacy goals and strategic partnerships are hidden behind most foreign aid. Despite framing foreign aid as development driven, Williams (2020) reveals that countries provide aid for a variety of reasons. For security reasons, aid may be provided to prevent a friendly country from falling under the influence of an unfriendly one. This was the case during the Cold War rivalry between the USA and the USSR in Africa. Today, the USA, European Union, and many other rich countries provide military aid to African countries to fight Islamic terrorism and piracy, forces that threaten the stability of the world order, and economic development. Countries may also use foreign aid to earn diplomatic recognition and get support for their positions in international organisations; finance their export trade; spread their culture and language; and promote

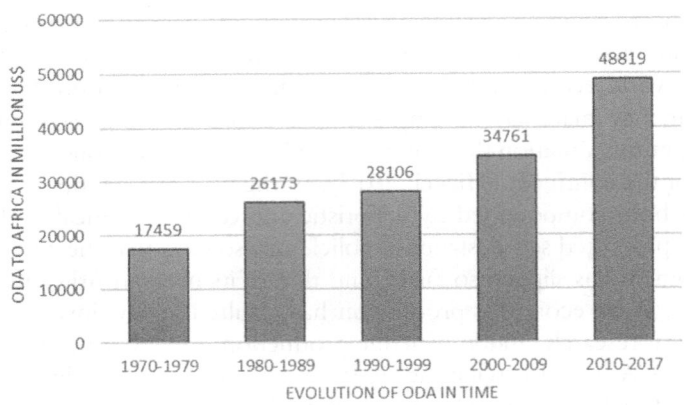

Fig. 5.1 The evolution of ODA to Africa over five decades. (Source: OECD (2022))

economic development and relieve the suffering caused by disease, war, disaster, and famine, among others. Figure 5.1 depicts the steady growth of ODA in Africa over five decades.

The ready availability of loans, grants, and humanitarian assistance to African countries from China, OECD, IMF, World Bank, European Union, and many other countries and organisations has weakened the ability or willingness of African leaders and politicians to exploit innovative alternative sources of financing for its development from better budgeting, the domestic capital market, remittances, and the reversal of capital flight among others (Kwakye, 2010). Debt, repayment, and servicing have unbalanced budgeting for social and economic development in Africa and further reinforced its dependency. Many countries are unable to execute the social components of their budgets because of debt servicing and repayment. Because of that, quite a few continental engagements at the level of the AU, including members' contributions, cannot be paid regularly. African countries look more to their richer counterparts in Europe, North America, and Asia for economic cooperation than to their African neighbours. This is reinforced by the continued strength of economic, social, and political ties between African countries and their former colonial masters.

Africa's colonial history has been exploited for the diplomatic advantage of former colonial masters in international organisations like the UN and its various agencies, as well as for the strategic interests of the members of the donor community such as the OECD. In assessing the performances of OECD countries in three aid areas (development gaps, global cooperation, and public-spiritedness), the Principled Aid Index (PAI) 2020 observed that major aid donors consistently ranked low in meeting development gaps and global cooperation dimensions but scored significantly higher in the aid-for-trade domain (Gulrajani, 2020). Aid for trade tends to achieve only narrow gains in the recipient community as cheap imports tend to weaken local production. France, for example, continues to focus most of its aid on Francophone Africa where it wields significant economic, social, and diplomatic influence (Gulrajani, 2020).

- *Multiple allegiances to regional economic groupings*

Added to the problem of shared external allegiances is the problem of membership in multiple regional economic groupings. Only 13 out of 53 African countries belong to only one regional economic grouping. These are Algeria, Cabo Verde, Liberia, Botswana, Lesotho, Malawi, Mozambique, Namibia, South Africa, Zambia, Zimbabwe, Egypt, Sao Tome, and Principe. The philosophy behind regional economic groupings is for them to constitute the foundation blocks of the AU by enhancing cooperation among African countries in these groups. Because of the plurality of group membership, scarce financial and material energies are dissipated by struggling to meet multiple targets. This is reflected in the poor quality of resources members contribute to the AU. This imperils the lofty health projects hatched by the AU in the past few years.

- *Recurrent Conflict*

Perhaps, only Asia witnesses armed conflicts on the frequency and scale close to Africa today (Buhaug & Rudolfsen, 2015). Armed conflict in Africa takes multiple forms: civil wars, sectarian violence, territorial disputes, and transnational terrorism. Violent conflict displaces populations, destroys communities and livelihoods, and breaks health systems. Levy and Sidel (2016) indicate that not only do healthcare delivery systems suffer during violent conflicts, but health-supporting infrastructures such as water, sanitation, communication, transportation, power, food production, and supply systems also do. Sato (2019) reports that the ongoing Boko Haram insurgency in north-eastern Nigeria has had a significant effect on the annual inoculation of children where more than 40 percent of residents within 10 km of a conflict are likely not to receive a vaccine.

If Africa must be ready for the heightened risks of frequent and virulent viral pandemics in the future, the AU must revisit its funding strategies which till date have been disproportionately reliant on external sources. Member states must become more committed and pay their dues regularly to the union. In 2016, the 27th African Union Summit held in Kigali implemented a 0.2 percent levy on eligible imports to be collected by each member to boost the finances of the African Union. The taxable base of the AU import levy is the value of eligible goods originating from a non-Member State imported into the territory of a Member State to be consumed in the Member State. The revenue collected under the import levy is then remitted in accordance with each Member State's approved assessed contribution including the Peace Fund. The implementation of the levy started in 2017 to finance 100 percent of the AU's operational budget, 75 percent programme budget, and 25 percent budget of the peace support operations of the African Union as well as any other expenditure of the Union that may be determined by the Assembly. Unfortunately, not all countries are collecting this import tax. As of 2018, only 16 countries of the 53 members of the AU were collecting this revenue. This speaks to the precariousness of the finances of the AU and its ability to deliver the objectives it set for the continent in its constitutive act of 2000. Without strong internal financing sources, the armada of institutions which have been created in the past five years to enhance disease prevention and health promotion will be unable to deliver its mandates.

REFERENCES

Alden, C., & Dunst, C. (2020). COVID-19: African and the African Union. LSE, Department of International Relations. https://www.lse.ac.uk/international-relations/centres-and-units/global-south-unit/covid-19-regional-responses/africa-and-covid-19.

AU. (2020). Financing the Union: Towards the financial autonomy of the African Union. Status Report-An update. Version Four.

AU. (2021). Treaty for the establishment of the African Medicines Agency (AMA) enters into force. https://au.int/en/pressreleases/20211109/treaty-establishment-african-medicines-agency-ama-enters-force.

AU. (n.d.). Division for health, nutrition and population. *African Union*. https://au.int/pt/node/32895

AU/Africa CDC. (n.d.). Disease information. *Centre for Disease Control and Prevention*. https://africacdc.org/disease/.

AUC. (2015). Africa health strategy 2016–2030. *African Union Commission.* https://au.int/sites/default/files/documents/30357-doc-final_ahs_strategy_formatted.pdf.

Buhaug, H., & Rudolfsen, I. (2015). A climate conflict? Technical Report, PRIO/ Conflict Trends. www.prio.org/ConflictTrends

Fonn, S. (2018). Research-intensive universities in Africa? A model of how to build them. *The Conversation.* https://phys.org/news/2018-09-research-intensive-universities-africa.html

Hickel, J (2017). The divide. A brief guide to global inequality and its solutions. London, Penguin Random House.

Gallup, J. L., & Sachs, J. D. (2001). The intolerable burden of malaria: A new look at the numbers. In J. G. Breman, A. Egan, & G. T. Keusch (Eds.), *Supplement to 64(1) of the American journal of tropical medicine and hygiene.* American Society of Tropical Medicine and Hygiene. https://www.ncbi.nlm. nih.gov/books/NBK2622/

Gulrajani, N. (2020). Principled aid index 2020. Working Papers. https://odi. org/en/publications/principled-aid-index-2020/.

Kwakye, J. K. (2010). Overcoming Africa's addiction to foreign aid: A look at some financial engineering to mobilise other resources. The Institution of Economic Affairs. https://www.africaportal.org/publications/overcoming-africas-addiction-to-foreign-aid-a-look-at-some-financial-engineering-to-mobilize-other-resources/.

Levy, B. S., & Sidel, V. W. (2016). Documenting the effects of armed conflict on population health. *Annual Review of Public Health, 37*, 205–218. https://doi. org/10.1146/annurev-publhealth-032315-021913

Lukwa, A. T., Mawoyo, R., Zablon, K. N., Siya, A., & Alaba, O. (2019). Effect of malaria on productivity in a workplace: The case of a banana plantation in Zimbabwe. *Malaria Journal, 18,* 390. https://doi.org/10.1186/ s12936-019-3021-6

Mahase, E. (2020). Coronavirus: Covid-19 has killed more people than SARS and MERS combined, despite lower case fatality rate. *BMJ, 368,* m641. https:// doi.org/10.1136/bmj.m641

Ndi, H. N., Ndi, R. A., Bang, H. N., Mbah, M. F., & Ndzo, J. A. (2021). Health and economic imperatives for households in the context of the anti-Covid-19 strategy in Cameroon. The case of Yaounde. *Journal of Humanities and Applied Social Sciences, 3*(5), 356–375. https://doi.org/10.1108/JHASS-01-2021-0016

OECD. (2022). Financing for sustainable development. https://www.oecd.org/ dac/financing-sustainable-development/.

Olufadewa, I. I., Adesina, M. A., & Ayorinde, T. (2020). From Africa to the world: Reimagining Africa's research capacity and culture in the global knowledge economy. *Journal of Global Health, 10*(1). https://doi.org/10.7189/jogh.10.010321

PEPFAR (2020). PEPFAR Latest Global Results: https://www.state.gov/wp-content/uploads/2020/12/PEPFAR-Latest-Results-Fact-Sheet-2020.pdf

Pharatlhatlhe, K., & Vanheukelom, J. (2019). Financing the African Union on mindsets and money. Discussion Paper No. 240. https://ecdpm.org/application/files/7216/6074/7083/DP240-Financing-the-African-Union-on-mindsets-and-money.pdf.

PMI. (2022). Cameroon Malaria operational plan FY 2022. President's Malaria Initiative. https://www.pmi.gov/where-we-work/cameroon/.

Sato, R. (2019). Effect of armed conflict on vaccination: Evidence from the Boko Haram insurgency in north-eastern Nigeria. *Conflict and Health, 13*(49). https://doi.org/10.1186/s13031-019-0235-8

Tatarsky, A., Aboobakar, S., Cohen, J. M., Gopee, N., Bheecarry, A., Moonasar, D., Phillips, A. A., Kahn, J. G., Moonen, B., Smith, D. L., & Sabot, O. (2011). Preventing the reintroduction of Malaria in Mauritius: *PLoS ONE, 6*(9). https://doi.org/10.1371/journal.pone.0023832.

UNAIDS. (2014). 90-90-90: An ambitious treatment target to end the AIDS pandemic. *The Joint United Nations Programme on HIV and AIDS.* https://www.unaids.org/sites/default/files/media_asset/90-90-90_en.pdf.

UNAIDS. (2016, May 27). Intellectual property and access to health technologies—questions and answers, *UNAIDS.* https://www.unaids.org/en/resources/documents/2016/JC2820.

UNAIDS. (2017, July 3). Africa Union endorses major new initiative to end AIDS. *The Joint United Nations Programme on HIV and AIDS.* https://www.unaids.org/en/resources/presscentre/pressreleaseandstatementarchive/2017/july/20170704_africanunion#:~:text=endorsed%20two%20major-,GENEVA%2C%20ADDIS%20ABABA%2C%203%20July%202017%E2%80%94African%20heads%20of,workers%20across%20Africa%20by%202020.

UNGA. (2001). Declaration of commitment on HIV/AIDS. Resolution adopted by the General Assembly, 62nd Special session, Agenda 7 (A/RES/S-26/2). https://documents-dds-ny.un.org/doc/UNDOC/GEN/N01/434/84/PDF/N0143484.pdf?OpenElement.

UNGA. (2006). Political declaration on HIV/AIDS. Resolution adopted by the General Assembly, 60th Session, Agenda item 45 (A/RES/60/262). https://hivlanguagecompendium.org/pdf/2006-A-RES-60-262%20PD%20on%20HIV-AIDS.pdf.

UNGA. (2009). Global health and foreign policy. Resolution adopted by the General Assembly, 63rd Session, Agenda item 44 (A/RES/63/33). https:// digitallibrary.un.org/record/642456?ln=en.

USFDA. (2018). Anthrax. US Food and Drug Administration. https://www.fda. gov/vaccines-blood-biologics/vaccines/anthrax#:~:text=The%20mortal-ity%20rates%20from%20anthrax,that%20is%2080%25%20or%20higher.

WHO. (2021). HIV/AIDS. https://www.afro.who.int/health-topics/hivaids.

WHO. (2022). Malaria. World Health Organisation. https://www.who.int/ news-room/fact-sheets/detail/malaria

WHO. (n.d.). Cholera dashboards. https://www.who.int/activities/supporting-cholera-outbreak-response/interactive-summary-visuals-ofcholera-data-officially-reported-to-who-since-2000

WHO. (n.d.). Ebola disease. https://africacdc.org/disease/.

Williams. (2020, November 5). Victoria. Foreign aid. *Encyclopaedia Britannica.* https://www.britannica.com/topic/foreign-aid.

CHAPTER 6

Violent Conflict, Diplomacy, and Health in Africa

Humphrey Ngala Ndi

INTRODUCTION

Violent conflict is a common occurrence in Africa. As such, the relatively poor health status of African populations does not always result from weak health systems, and inaccessibility to health services, but also the result of violent conflict that disproportionately affects health infrastructure and personnel when and where they occur. In 2021, the Africa Center for Strategic Studies estimated that 32 million Africans were living away from their homes having been forcibly displaced by conflict and repression. Up to 88 per cent of these people originated in only ten of Africa's 54 countries. Virtually every country in the world has experienced a conflict in its history. In Africa, two types of violent conflicts stand out. These are border conflicts (inter-state) and internal conflicts (intra-state). While intrastate conflicts are more violent, intense, shorter in duration, and create the most suffering, deaths, and refugee in African populations, the inter-state

H. N. Ndi (✉)
High Commission for the Republic of Cameroon in London, London, UK

University of Yaounde I, Yaounde, Cameroon

© The Author(s), under exclusive license to Springer Nature   121
Switzerland AG 2023
H. N. Ndi et al. (eds.), *Health Diplomacy in Africa*, Studies in
Diplomacy and International Relations,
https://doi.org/10.1007/978-3-031-41249-3_6

ones are often less dramatic, generating fewer deaths and refugees but are more protracted.

African inter-state conflicts generally revolve around issues of transboundary resources including farmlands, and transboundary tribes and ethnic groups, which render the implementation of colonial and postcolonial boundary agreements difficult. While inter-state conflicts may be common in Africa, the violent ones are few following the definition of the Uppsala Conflict Data Program (UCDP). This suggests that 25 deaths in battle in a calendar year meet the criteria of a conflict. This suggestion ignores the fact that not all conflicts become violent because states may disagree over boundaries but prefer to seek the adjudication of an international court or favour the use of preventive diplomacy where international organisations like the African Union or the United Nations seek to restore trust between the conflicting parties through negotiation and compromise.

Ikome (2012) of the Institute for Security Studies notes that more than half of African countries have been involved in some form of boundary-related conflict since the 1950s. Colonial boundaries agreed upon at the Berlin Conference in 1884–1885 had no regard for the social fabric of African societies, practically tearing some apart and assigning them to different colonial possessions. Astronomical and mathematical lines used as boundaries are very abstract and difficult to implement.

Intra-state conflicts in Africa generally result from poor leadership or governance, though this itself is tacitly linked to international meddling facilitated by the fragile structure the African state inherited from colonisation. In a depiction of the French stands towards the decolonisation of its African colonies, Smith and Jeppesen (2017) and Hodgkin (1956) show how General Charles de Gaulle, the French president, from 1959 to 1969 perceived Africa's role in the post-Second World War recovery of the French economy after the defeat of Nazi Germany. It was an absolute position for him that the colonial empire would remain French as the War had proven the value of the empire to France for post-War recovery and he was determined to ensure the legitimacy and security of French colonies. To Charles de Gaulle, the end of the so-called civilising mission in the colonies excluded any idea of autonomy and the possibility of evolution outside the French bloc. It also excluded the eventual establishment of self-government, even in a distant future where independence for Africa simply meant European powers accommodating adjustments and compromises in the face of African nationalism. This stance is reflected in the importance of colonial factors in fashioning contemporary economic, political, and social developments in Africa including the emergence of regional political conflicts. True to their policy of keeping their African colonial possession within the French bloc, the nature of the French-Africa relations after independence kept the former African territories structurally dependent on France economically, fiscally, politically, diplomatically, and culturally (Joseph, 1978). This was achieved through the imposition of the so-called Cooperation Agreements the French signed with the newly independent African countries. Independence failed to sever the umbilical cord between African states and France. The cord is exploited to maintain those local elite permitted by France to inherit legal sovereignty in power (ibid.) and evict those with whom they have no favour.

These arrangements continue to cause internal poverty in African countries, entrenching inequality in wealth distribution, and perpetrating predatory governance, political corruption, rampant civil strife, and ethnic conflicts.

Fabricius (2019) suggests that intra-state conflicts in Africa result from inequality in society, entrenched poverty, undemocratic behaviours especially electoral fraud, gross violations of human rights, the proliferation of illegal arms, the fragility of the state, government corruption, uncontrolled exploitation of natural resources, climate change, neo-colonialist connections, and illegitimate African leadership. Worthy of note is also the quest for unfettered access to Africa's mineral wealth which has pushed some countries in Europe and North America to undermine independent-minded African leaders who have wanted to exercise firm control over their African resources for the benefit of their peoples.

African countries endowed with rare natural resources like oil, gas, and gemstones have often been deeply embroiled in the devastating conflict. Ross (2004) posits that Oil increases the likelihood of conflict particularly the fight to secede from the main polity; but lootable resources like gemstones and drugs do not trigger conflict although they are more likely to lengthen existing ones.

Inter-state conflicts may sometimes lead to a breakdown of diplomatic relations between the states involved, preventing them from cooperating over transborder projects like disease surveillance, cross-border health data sharing, sharing security information, fighting smuggling and piracy, and the trade in contraband goods. On the other hand, intra-state conflicts in Africa tend to create more impact not only in the country of the conflict but also across international borders. Mengisteab (2003/2004) observes that intra-state conflicts may cause states to fail to trigger severe economic dislocation and disruption in the provision of public services. By generating large waves of internally displaced people and refugees, intra-state conflicts have proven to exacerbate the spread of infectious diseases like HIV/AIDS, and cholera and have also weakened health systems.

STRUCTURAL CAUSES OF INTRA-STATE CONFLICT IN AFRICA

Mengisteab (2003/2004) encapsulates the structural causes of intra-state conflicts in Africa under four related points:

The nature of the post-independence African state is a primordial centrifugal and conflictual factor. Many African states are made up of highly ethnically unconsolidated groups of people who pay more allegiance to their communities, traditions, and cultures than the state. This character neither makes the state an overarching organisation nor does it enhance the inclusivity of all citizens in the polity as governments often operate a leadership and infrastructural apparatus unaccountable to the citizenry. Hegre (2000) and Ross (2004) have suggested a causal link between a government's lack of accountability and the likelihood of civil strife. The 'strongman' politics, so common of the African political landscape is essentially predatory. Where the head of state is also head of the judiciary, army, police, and bureaucracy, coercive and violent means are habitually used to redistribute income from the masses to the ruling class, which wealth is in turn recycled to prop the 'strongman' from falling, while he presides over the failure of the state. In this system, African leaders not only engage in gross corruption and mismanagement of state resources but also behave as if they owned the state to use it the way they want. The post-independence African state has neither developed an inclusive system of governance nor has it distinguished itself as a neutral apparatus capable of acting fairly for its citizens.

The proto-colonial nature of the post-colonial African state has prevented Africans from evolving their own personalities based on their unique circumstances. African political elite inherited the apparatus of the colonial state and maintained its predatory characteristics instead of reconstituting it to ensure that it advanced the interest of its citizens. The bureaucracies inherited from the colonialists were expanded and entrenched which reinforced their dependency on the former colonial powers. The emergence of a neo-colonial political culture also entrenched predatory practices. Joseph (1978) illustrates how Léopold Sédar Senghor and Houphouet-Boigny were strongly impressed by the ideals of the Franco-African Community, and by their opportunity to participate in French governments and devise laws for this community just like their metropolitan colleagues. Gabon's first president Leon M'ba had wished to make his country a French overseas territory so that all Gabonese will also hold French nationality (Britannica, 2022). The close relationship between France and her ex-African colonies has continued and provides a framework for the domination of these territories through loyal and faithful African interlocutors. In most French African colonies, independence was not granted to those who wanted and fought for it. Rather, it was granted to loyalists. As such the seeds of conflict were built into the foundation stones of many African countries.

Another important cause of intra-state conflicts in Africa is the privatisation of the state and the inability of early leaders to bring it under the control of citizens. Shortly after independence, many countries abolished multiparty politics, putting an end to exogenous political competition. From thence, the head of state wielded wide-ranging discretionary powers manipulating it not to benefit the people they rule over, but as bait for those seeking political favours, and while doing so, setting the price of their political loyalty (Bates, 2008). The social contract between the governing class and the governed was breached because political power lost consensual legitimacy. The 'strongman' controlled the electoral process in the one-party state, where voting for the head of state and the House of Representatives was mandatory and coercive. The Africa Center for Strategic Studies posits that the utter lack of legitimacy and accountability reflecting the inability of political systems to accommodate participation, contestation, and power-sharing are at the root of many of Africa's deadly conflicts.

The demise of the USSR and the end of the Cold War in 1991 marked the beginning of a unipolar world led by the USA and her European allies. Using democratic reforms as a condition for assistance and cooperation, the USA, the European Union, the World Bank, and the IMF compelled many African countries to open the political space by embracing participation and political competition. Multipartyism was reintroduced and competitive elections were held for the first time in more than 30 years in many countries. Presidential terms were often limited for many countries. Twenty years down the line, there have been strong reversals in democratic gains on the continent. Not only have the democratic processes become corrupted but term limits have been lifted in many countries allowing the heads of state to consolidate their grips on power despite the often-popular outcry for alternation. Table 6.1 summarises the responses to presidential term limits in Africa since the reintroduction of multiparty democracy.

Table 6.1 Presidential term limits in Africa

Presidential term	Number of countries
No term limits	9
Limit not yet met by any president	9
Limit modified or eliminated	16
Limit retained after an attempt to modify or eliminate	6
Limit respected with leader leaving office	14

Source: Africa Center for Strategic Studies (2021)

There has been a reversal in participation and alternation of power in 16 countries making the continent one where more than 12 presidents have ruled for more than twenty uninterrupted years. The Africa Center for Strategic Studies observes that 8 of the 11 African countries facing conflict and instability have not instituted presidential term limits, and two are under unconstitutional military rule (Siegle, 2021 and Siegle & Cook, 2020). Whereas 9 of Africa's 16 autocracies are experiencing conflict, none of the continent's democracies are in conflict. In 2020, about 29 million people in Africa were forcibly displaced from their homes. Over 72 per cent of this number originated in 10 countries, 9 of them autocratic and one a flawed democracy. As such, reversing the trends in forced displacement in Africa will require that the primary causes (repressive governance and conflict) are deliberately addressed.

The use of the tribal or ethnic card to intimidate or criminalise opponents and incite public anger against them is so common in Africa. As a means of extending their stay in power, autocratic leaders are unable to maintain neutrality in public affairs, choosing rather manipulate ethnicity to accentuate division and alienate or weaken their opponents.

The use of tribes to foster political gain on the continent can be traced back to the colonial period when colonialists promoted tribal rivalries and jealousies as part of a \divide-and-rule strategy to weaken strong ethnic groups capable of undermining colonial authority or pitting such groups against each other. In such ways, they became arbiters of peace and were accepted by the belligerent parties as peacemakers. The English regularly set the Kikuyus and the Luo of Kenya whom they viewed as dangerous to their colonial interests because of their vast populations; in Cameroon, the French used the ethnic card to fight and destroy the *Union des Populations du Cameroun* (UPC) nationalist political party which refused independence for Cameroon on the terms the administering colonial power had proposed for the territory. To raze out the most ardent supporters of this party, an ethnic colouration was given to the ferocious war against UPC nationalists in the Bamileke and Bassa territories of the country described in the most deceitful terms by the colonial French administrators and its Cameroonian proxies as the pacification of the territory from guerrilla insurgents (Deltombe et al., 2016). Similarly, the divide between the Tutsis and Hutus in Rwanda and Burundi was accentuated by the colonialists. In Rwanda, the Belgians had a policy of supporting the minority Tutsis by requiring that all local chiefs be Tutsis, to the resentment of the majority Hutus. In the country's first elections at independence in 1961, the Hutus easily won and the regime that followed was staunchly nationalist, sowing the seeds for the eventual premeditated attempt to cleanse the country of Tutsis. This eventually happened in the 1994 Rwandan genocide in which over 800,000 Tutsis and moderate Hutus were slain by Hutu extremists.

No African country was spared the colonialist use of the tribe in divide-and-rule tactics. Unfortunately, post-independence African leaders have continued to use it to seek or consolidate political power. The problem with advancing the economic and political interests of one tribe against others in a country is that it internalises the conflictual culture of retribution and resistance, in the politicians and populations of other tribes when power slips into their hands.

When violent conflict erupts in any society or country, the first casualty is usually the social fabric and infrastructure. As people are displaced towards more secure zones or countries, transport arteries become unsafe, and peacemakers call for restraint, healthcare units suffer from a lack of essential medical supplies and staff. In the destinations, similar infrastructure comes under unsustainable pressure and a decline in the quality of care and personal as well as environmental hygiene with an attendant heightened risk of infectious disease outbreak ensues. Given that no internal violent conflict can be contained within national frontiers streams of refugees flooding neighbouring countries are often common.

In the context of this book, the Tutsi and Hutu refugee crisis and the resultant inter-militia violence in the eastern Democratic Republic of Congo will provide the basis for the discussion of the health diplomacy implications of an internal conflict with a transborder element.

KINSTATE DYNAMICS IN THE EASTERN DEMOCRATIC
REPUBLIC OF CONGO CRISIS

Colonialism created artificial and arbitrary boundaries in Africa that tore apart nations or ethnic groups and placed them within newly found states on the continent. In the process, the phenomenon of kinstates or groups developed. Waterbury (2020) defines a kinstate as a state that represents the majority nation of a transborder ethnic group whose members reside in neighbouring territories. As indicated earlier, arbitrarily drawn colonial boundaries created many kinstates in Africa. A few outstanding examples include Nigeria whose Yoruba population is also found in Benin and Togo; Kenya whose Luo ethnic group also exists in Tanzania; the Democratic Republic of the Congo whose Lunda population also exists in Angola; South Africa whose Zulu population is also found in Lesotho, Eswatini, and Botswana, and perhaps Rwanda and Burundi as the most outstanding examples which will serve for illustrating the health implications of conflictual transborder kin relations in Africa.

Rwanda and Burundi provide a unique example of kinstates to each other created by the colonial enterprise. Both countries are composed of about 85 per cent Hutus, 14 per cent Tutsis, and 1 per cent Twa (pygmies). They are thus kinstates to each other. Both countries have significant populations in the Kivu region of eastern Congo which unfortunately have been a main factor in the decades-long instability of the region. Of North Kivu's 4 million inhabitants, 50 per cent are the indigenous Nande; 30 per cent are Hutus; and the remaining 20 per cent are Hunde, Nyanga, and Tutsis, the latter being settlers (Lawson et al., 2010).

The migration of Banyarwanda (Tutsis and Hutus from Rwanda) was actively promoted by the Belgians in the late nineteenth and early twentieth centuries when the territory of Ruanda-Urundi, a former German colony, was passed unto Belgian control in the Mandate system as territories of the League of Nations in the Versailles Peace Treaty that ended the Second World War. The territories later became the Trust Territories of the United Nations Organisation, when the League of Nations ceased to exist in 1946. The first major wave of migration in the early twentieth century was caused by overpopulation and famine in Rwanda which pushed them to seek labour jobs in agricultural activities in North Kivu. They were generally treated more favourably by the Belgians at the expense of the natives, sowing the early seeds of ethnic tensions that have persisted in the region to date. In 1960, there were already about 200,000 Rwandan phones in the DRC (Jacquemot, 2010). The Rwandan genocide of 1994 generated a second important wave of Hutu and Tutsi refugee movements into North and South Kivu. In 2000, about two million Rwandan Hutus fled to the DRC whose eastern borders have historically been porous (Venugopalan, 2016).

Among them were Hutus who had perpetrated the genocide and were escaping from the Rwandan Patriotic Front (RPF), a Tutsi-led rebel group that was poised to take over the country. In Kivu, the newly arrived Hutus who included ex-Armed Forces of Rwanda (ex-FAR) and the *Interahamwe* (Hutu paramilitary group that participated in the Rwandan genocide) easily joined the ranks of local Hutu militias to launch attacks on Congolese Tutsis, perceived to be sympathetic to the RPF which was advancing on Kigali. They also launched cross-border attacks against Rwanda, Burundi, and Uganda.

This refugee movement significantly disrupted the demographic balance in the region, much to the distaste of Congolese authorities. Pressure on the land and the essentials of life like water, wood, and fertile land also triggered conflict between the Tutsis and Hutus in the Kivu region. From the 1990s, the discovery of valuable minerals like coltan and cassiterite in Northern Kivu, highly sought after by electronic companies and other industrialists, further compounded the situation in the region. Hutu and Tutsi militias all scrambled for these minerals to fund their activities.

The Congolese army's inability to purge the region of the paramilitaries groups and to protect ethnic minorities with cross-border links to Rwanda, Burundi, and Uganda dragged these countries to intervene in the region. Furthermore, the Mobutu government's decision to strip the *Kinyarwanda-speaking* populations (*Banyarwanda* and *Banyamulenge*) of Congolese nationality because of their disruptive activities heightened fears of ethnic cleansing. The *Banyamulenge* refer exclusively to Congolese Tutsis concentrated in South Kivu, and the *Banyarwanda* refers to the Tutsi, Hutu, and Batwa people concentrated in both North and south Kivu.

In response to President Mobutu, the Banyamulenge launched preemptive strikes against the Zairian national army and Hutu refugee camps in September 1996. In solidarity, the Rwandan army entered the conflict in support of the Banyamulenge, but also to rout out remnants of the ex-members of the Rwanda Armed Forces (FAR) mainly Hutus militias who had participated in the genocide and were still using eastern Congo to launch attacks against Rwanda. The Ugandan army also entered eastern

Congo because it was being used by anti-Museveni forces. In this chaos, Rwanda and Uganda engaged in pillaging the resources of eastern Congo.

Seizing this opportunity, Laurent Kabila, Mobutu's long-time enemy and rebel leader, swung the Alliance of Democratic Forces for the Liberation of Congo-Zaire, supported principally by Rwanda, and Uganda, to defend against the possibility of anti-Tutsi attacks. This eventually led to the overthrow of Mobutu in 1997. Having been aided by foreign forces to gain power, Kabila was rather a Rwandan puppet and his attempt to assert his power as a sovereign leader by ejecting all foreign forces who helped him gain power but who were now undermining his authority cost him Rwandan friendship and eventually led to his demise in 2001.

Under the guise of preventing ethnic cleansing and fighting anti-Rwandan and Ugandan forces in the Congo, these countries have systematically pillaged the resources of the latter through proxy militias who are not ready to give up their activities, especially in the context of a security void characteristic of failed states for which the DRC is one. From 1997 to 1998, for example, Uganda's diamond exports increased 12 times, while Congo's exports of the same mineral declined by 50 per cent (ibid.). With the failure of the DRC to secure its borders and the multiplicity of splinter militias funding their activities from the exploitation of the country's minerals, rivalry and violence became a permanent feature of this region.

There are over 120 militia groups operating in the Kivu region and violence is a common feature of life in the region. For many years, the tactical and strategical involvement of Rwanda and Uganda in the eastern Congo crisis has frozen cooperation among these countries and rendered a negotiated settlement difficult. Uganda claims that the Allied Democratic Forces (ADF), a Uganda rebel coalition that pays allegiance to the Islamic State and is responsible for a string of bombings in Kampala is operating from North Kivu and the Ituri. Rwanda on its part sees the continued operation of the predominantly Hutu ex-Armed Forces of Rwanda, now the *Interahamwe* as a major perpetual threat. Thus, a weak Congolese army and the security vacuum created in eastern Congo are perceived as a threat to President Paul Kagame's regime especially.

The Sun City Peace Agreement of 2003 after the inter-Congolese dialogue that brought together some of the warring parties in the country was broken shortly after it was signed by Laurent Nkunda, a Congolese Tutsi claiming to protect the Tutsi from attack by the Congolese people in North Kivu. On January 2009, Nkunda, a Rwandan proxy was arrested by

Rwandan forces on the Uganda–Congo border, to ease reconciliation between Nkunda's Tutsi militia (The National Congress for the Defence of the People—CNDP) and the Congolese Defence Forces signalling diplomatic rapprochement between the DRC and Rwanda. Perhaps, the neutralisation of Nkunda was simply Rwanda's attempt to cleanse its international image as an aggressor without genuinely committing to withdraw covert support to Tutsi militias in the eastern DRC. This is because it withdrew support from the CNDP probably because of its internal discords that could no longer serve Rwandan interests only to pass it on to the newly formed and more formidable M23 Congolese Tutsi rebel group.

The arrival of Felix Tshisekedi in 2019 momentarily brought hope of peace in eastern Congo when he and President Kagame of Rwanda signed a bilateral agreement on investments, trade, and the joint exploitation of gold to set the pace for the restoration of peace in the Kivu region. However, in 2020, a UN expert group reported the presence of Rwanda Defence Forces in North Kivu, and in 2021, an RDF incursion met with fire from the Congolese army (FARDC) (UNSC, 2020). Relations between Rwanda and the DRC further deteriorated when on February 8, 2022, President Kagame seemed to insinuate that anti-Rwanda forces were operating from within the DRC. "All eyes are on Congo. We are focused there because of the armed groups based there that threaten us. When someone crosses a red line, we don't ask anybody for permission to intervene. To whoever wants war from us, we give it to him" (Reyntjens, 2022). On March 28, 2022, elements of the M23 attacked Congolese army positions in several strategic places in North Kivu.

The security dynamics caused by two transborder ethnic groups (the Tutsi) loyal to the current Rwandan government, and the other (Hutus) hostile to it, operating in North Kivu, represent a perennial threat to Kagame's regime. The threat is so apparent because, Goma, the capital of North Kivu is only 162 km from Kigali or 3.5 hours by car. Thus, the Rwandan Defence Forces are wary of the menace that a formidable Hutu militia operating from Kivu can pose to the Rwandan state. The mineral wealth of the Congo region of Kivu has also been attractive to neighbouring Rwanda and Uganda which covertly exploit it through the militias they support. On the other hand, the strong loyalties shown by the Tutsi militias to their kin state—Rwanda, make it difficult for them to be integrated into Congolese society. The security situation in the Kivu region continues to befuddle the international community and hopes for a lasting solution are still out of sight. Maybe, the recent decision by the East African Community (EAC) to send a joint force to combat armed groups in the region is signalling hope for the region (Russo, 2022). However, the exclusion of Rwanda forces from the mission and the undefined relationship between the EAC military expedition and the UN Peace Keeping Force (MONUSCO operating in the region) may undermine the effort.

In the decades that this conflict has lasted, the main casualties have been the population, displaced and deprived of social development. The failure of a diplomatic solution within the context of the Great Lakes region continues to inflict a devastating toll on the health of the populations of the Kivu region, rendered helpless and suspicious of voluntary workers in the face of deadly infectious diseases like Cholera, HIV/AIDS, and the Ebola Virus Disease (EVD).

THE NEXUS OF VIOLENT CONFLICT, DIPLOMACY, AND HEALTH

Violent conflict, health, and diplomacy operate in an intimate nexus. Both inter-state and intra-state conflicts may become violent when diplomacy fails. They orchestrate dramatic health problems and weaken the social, economic, and political barriers against the spread of infectious disease, as food production and healthcare systems collapse. In general, diplomacy and health protection and promotion decline when violent conflict ensues. Diplomacy is largely contingent on the existence of a liberal democratic culture, a favourable condition for political, economic, and social advancement, where conflicting parties are willing to entertain compromises over the red lines that led to conflict. Unfortunately, conventional military operations and those of insurgent militias in a conflict scenario often target essential infrastructure like water and electricity plants, and schools and hospitals as a strategy of deliberately hurting civilians to stir public opinion against an opposing party in the conflict. Even when wars have ended, health risks such as contaminated water, dangerous landmines, undetonated bombs, grenades, and food shortages have persisted for a long. What is now known as 'green famine' refers to food shortages in places with fertile, cultivable land abandoned to landmines (Loretti, 1997; Kalipeni & Oppong, 1998). Worst still, criminality and trauma continue because it takes a long to completely get rid of war weapons circulating in the population, as well as disarming and demobilising splinter militias,

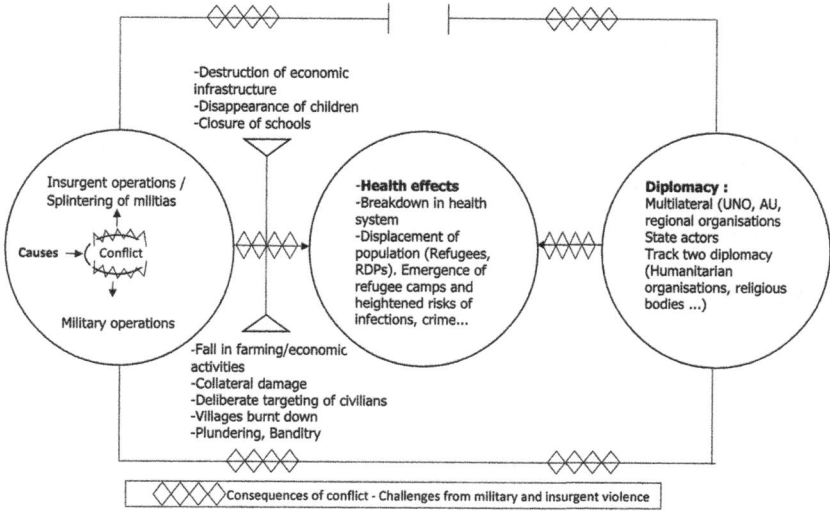

Fig. 6.1   The nexus between violent conflict, health, and diplomacy

common in protracted conflicts. Figure 6.1 illustrates the nexus between conflict, health, and diplomacy.

Loretti (1997), Kalipeni and Oppong (1998), Venugopalan (2016), Murray et al. (2002), and Njenga et al. (2006) among many others present a summary of some of the implications of diplomatic disputes and violent conflicts on health and disease. In general, societies in conflict experience a disruption of livelihood and healthcare delivery systems; poor sanitation, overcrowding, and food shortages; decline in reproductive healthcare and disease prevention; and trauma and mental health.

Conflict disrupts social life and wreaks havoc on the fragile health systems in sub-Saharan Africa. In protracted conflicts like the one in Angola (1975–2002), health units were destroyed, and the supply of essential health equipment was disrupted. Loretti (1997) notes that in the close to thirty years of conflict, the population of Luanda grew rapidly as the country sides became insecure. Consequently, the disproportion between the population and the supply of basic services like water and sanitation made cholera endemic in the city. Mobutu's support to the Angolan rebels of the National Union for the Total Independence of Angola (UNITA) movement made a regional diplomatic and humanitarian response to the effects of the war difficult. Child malnutrition in Angola reached 50 per cent (Kalipeni & Oppong, 1998), while the number of missing children rose to 200,000 in 1994 (Loretti, 1997). Levy and Sidel (2016) indicate that not only healthcare delivery systems suffer during violent conflicts. Health-supporting infrastructures such as water, sanitation, communication, transportation, power, food production, and supply systems also do (Sato, 2019) reports that the ongoing Boko Haram insurgency in north-eastern Nigeria has had a significant effect on the annual inoculation of children where more than 40 per cent of residents within 10 km of a conflict are likely not to receive a vaccine.

Violent conflict can affect health cooperation significantly because it scares off international emergency and humanitarian non-governmental organisations whose activities suffer in the backlash of population displacements. Since the start of its mission to create a caliphate in West Africa, the Boko Haram Islamic sect has repeatedly launched onslaughts against humanitarian and health workers in north-eastern Nigeria, its stronghold. Ewang (2019), writing for Human Rights Watch, documents cases of lethal violence directed at health and humanitarian workers in this region. In 2013, the sect killed nine polio workers in Kano; in March 2018, it abducted and later executed two employees of the International Committee of the Red Cross; and in July 2019, the sect killed six humanitarian and health workers in Borno State. On July 23, 2020, BBC News reported the abduction and execution of five humanitarian and health workers representing four international non-governmental organisations in Borno State. The sect has waged a persistent violent war against multilateral cooperation marked by its 2011 attack of the UN main office in Abuja killing eighteen workers (Ewang, 2019), and the 2020 attack on a major humanitarian hub in Ngala, Borno State (BBC News, 2020). These attacks consistently jeopardize the ability of aid workers to stay and deliver assistance to people most in need in the remote areas of Borno State. Territorial disputes witness heightened border control and surveillance which may slow down or hamper cross-border disease control. There are currently thirty active conflicts in Africa where the health conditions described above are common.

The manifestations of poor sanitation, overcrowding, and food shortages are felt nowhere else as intensely as in refugee camps and among forcibly displaced populations. According to the United Nations High Commission for Refugees (UNHCR), Africa has over 30 million forcibly displaced persons (United Nations, n.d.). Of this figure, 72 per cent are internally displaced or asylum seekers simply wanting to get out of harm's way in conflict-torn countries. Life in a refugee camp is a gamble and survival rates vary depending on the social and infrastructural capabilities of the recipient countries. Measles and cholera are among the most common diseases in these camps. In June 1994, one of the worst cholera epidemics broke out in a one million Rwandan refugee camp in Goma, eastern Zaire (today the Democratic Republic of the Congo) and 12,000 perished according to the estimates of the UNHCR (Siddique, 1994). Another one followed in 1997 in a Rwandan refugee camp of 90,000 people.

The conflict in the eastern DRC, termed by some as 'Africa's World War' has claimed more than 5 million lives and merits closer attention to understand the geopolitical and strategic interests of regional powers involved in it.

Reproductive health and the control and prevention of HIV/AIDS often decline in conflict areas. Rape becomes rampant when law and order break down, and as women try to escape to safety, many are raped in transit, and the vulnerable conditions in refugee camps result in more rapes. The results are a degeneration in the mental health of those affected, unwanted pregnancies, and the spread of sexually transmitted diseases including HIV/AIDS (Mengisteab, 2003/2004). The selling of sex for food is a rampant phenomenon in refugee camps. Since these camps accommodate people from areas with different HIV/AIDS prevalence rates, mixing up as refugees inevitably increases the spread. In the absence of basic healthcare services including antenatal care, many maternal and infant mortality rates are significantly higher among refugees. In the case of the DRC, the conflict in the eastern border regions has pushed human development to a very low level. The poverty rate here is up to 84.7 per cent in South Kivu and 73 per cent in North Kivu, higher than the national average of 71 per cent. Primary school attendance rates have fallen to around 50 per cent and maternal and infant mortality rates are very high. Very few households are connected to potable water systems and even fewer to the electricity grid. Health services are very inadequate with ratios of one doctor per 27,700 and 24,000 inhabitants in South Kivu and North Kivu respectively (Venugopalan, 2016).

THE HEALTH IMPLICATIONS OF THE CONFLICT IN EASTERN CONGO

The conflict in the Kivu region of eastern Congo is nearly 30 years today. Because of its protracted nature, the damage to the healthcare system is almost permanent. Belligerent factions often target and destroy soft infrastructure like schools, hospitals, water, and electricity supply systems in the hope of getting quick concessions when people are pushed into rebellion. Looting and kidnapping of civilians (health workers, teachers, and civil society actors) are common. This provokes a deluge of refugees and internally displaced persons running away to safety. In the process the aged, children, and women suffer the most with many families losing their members. In cases like this, the voluntary sector has shown tenacity and resilience although its interventions are more relief-oriented than the enhancement of the healthcare delivery system. Because of persistent violence, heightened risk of death, and a high volume of internally displaced persons, dreadful gaps have been created in access to healthcare in eastern Congo particularly in reproductive health and maternal and child health services (Kadir et al., 2019).

In addition, the collection of health and demographic data which are crucial for policy making has remained limited, disjointed, and sporadic and can neither provide a short-term nor long-term picture of the health of the population of the region. With the involvement of regional powers (Uganda and Rwanda) at different stages in the conflict, a regional approach to combatting epidemics or pandemics is difficult. A frequently occurring disease in the DRC is the Ebola Virus Disease (EVD). Of the 36 major EVD outbreaks in Africa, since the first outbreak in 1972, 15 have occurred in the DRC, 6 in Uganda, and 3 in South Sudan. Since 1979, the outbreaks of EVD in the DRC have become increasingly more frequent. For this reason, the scare of the Ebola Virus Disease is real in the countries of the Great Lakes region of Africa. Whenever there is an outbreak in the DRC, Uganda or South Sudan, the neighbouring countries immediately roll out preventive measures which may be border closures or screening, and/or the vaccination of border populations. The September 2022 EVD outbreak in Uganda has triggered mass vaccinations in Rwanda with screening booths set up for travellers at the borders. An earlier and similar outbreak in North Kivu lasted longer than expected because of conflict promoted by the multiplicity of warring militias who often direct attacks on healthcare workers and the pervasive suspicion of government and international efforts (Gully, 2020). The United Nations Office for the Coordination of Humanitarian Affairs has documented the number of attacks directed at health workers in 2021 in the restive eastern region of the DRC. This is shown in Table 6.2.

In the absence of security in eastern Congo, the episodes, and frequencies of EVD have become longer and more intense. Because of the strained inter-state relations, EVD preventive measures lack the essential

Table 6.2 Violence against healthcare workers and health facilities in the eastern DRC

Killed	5
Kidnapped	27
Arrested	34
Injured	26
Assaulted	6
Attacks on health facilities	6
Forceful entry into health facilities	15
Looting, theft, robbery, and burglary of health supplies	63

Source: UNOCHA (2021)

cross-border element that can help countries which are centres of outbreak contain the virus within their borders. Rather, individual countries take measures that regulate and screen cross-border movements. The 2018 EVD outbreak in the DRC led to intensified cross-border collaboration among East African countries on disease surveillance and emergency preparedness. This provided an opportunity to create awareness among district leaders in their roles in implementing the International Health Regulations (IHR) of 2005. Consequently, the East African Integrated Disease Surveillance Network (EAIDSNet) convened a three-day cross-border meeting in Entebbe, Uganda, to enhance disease surveillance, emergency preparedness, and response in East Africa including the Democratic Republic of the Congo (DRC). With the accession of the DRC to membership of the East African Community (EAC) in 2022, it is hoped that greater concerted action in the region will galvanise the fight against virulent epidemics through the East African Community Contingency Plan for Epidemics due to communicable disease conditions and other relevant public health concerns 2018–2023 (Kajeguka, 2019). From a security perspective, the DRC's membership of the EAC may be a game changer in the crisis in the Kivu as that regional body has agreed to deploy troops to pacify the region. This scenario augurs well for disease surveillance and control.

The Great Lakes region of Africa and the Congo Basin are important *geogen* and the outbreaks of novel diseases especially of the zoonotic type are common. Table 6.3 presents a summary of disease outbreaks in East Africa over a seventeen-year period (2000–2017).

The Congo Basin and the Rift Valley ecosystems harbour pathogens and vectors that transmit numerous infectious diseases. Many of them are zoonotic in character and are triggered by man's tenacious search for natural resources in wild ecosystems settings with which contact has not been

Table 6.3   Disease outbreaks in the East African Community 2000–2017

Country	2000–2005	2006–2010	2011–2015	2016–2017
Burundi	Measles (2000)	–	Cholera (2012, 2013)	Cholera (2017)
Kenya	Meningitis (2000)	Rift Valley fever (2006–2007) Meningitis (2006) Cholera (2009)	Cholera (2010, 2014, 2015) Dengue (2011, 2013, 2014)	Cholera, Chikungunya, Anthrax (2017)
Rwanda	Meningitis (2000)	Pandemic influenza A (H1N1) (2009, 2010)	Cholera (2012	–
South Sudan	Anthrax (2005)	Rift Valley fever (2007) Highly pathogenic avian influenza (2006)	Anthrax (2014) Cholera (2014)	Cholera (2017)
Tanzania	Cholera (2002–2005)	Rift Valley fever (2006–2007) Measles (2006, 2007) Cholera (2006) Rabies (2009) new virus discovered in Tanzania in wild civet (Ikoma lyssavirus) Dengue (2010)	Cholera (2012, 2013, 2015) Hepatitis E (2013) Measles (2011) Dengue (2011, 2014) Plague (2011) Meningitis (2014) Anthrax (2012, 2014)	Cholera (Zanzibar 2016) Rabies (Zanzibar, 2015–2016)
Uganda	Measles (2001, 2002)	Yellow fever (2010) EVD (2007)	Meningitis (2012, 2014) EVD (2012) Marburg virus disease (2012) Crimean-Congo haemorrhagic fever (2013) Typhoid fever (2015)	Marburg (2017) RVF (2017) Crimean-Congo haemorrhagic fever (2017)
DRC[a]		EVD (2008–2009)	EVD (2014) Cholera (2011, 2015, 2017)	EVD (2017)

Source: Adapted from the East African Community regional contingency plan for epidemics due to communicable disease, conditions, and other events of public health concern 2018–2023

[a]The Democratic Republic of the Congo was admitted into the East African Community in 2022

established before. In the quest for mineral resources, timber and food, man gets into contact with many disease-carrying primates, animals, and birds capable of transmitting viruses and bacteria.

As the fourth most populous country in Africa with a population of 92 million in 2021, and an important *geogen* by virtue of the Congo Basin, the DRC which shares borders with nine other countries is an important epicentre of zoonotic infections and has the propensity to disperse them to its neighbours and to be a receptacle of infections from its neighbours too. The fragile security situation of the DRC makes it difficult for health workers to detect, respond, and control infectious disease outbreaks. It is critical that the response capacity of the DRC is strong enough to address public health threats within the country and prevent the spread of disease regionally and globally. Diplomacy is indispensable in this case and the African Union ought to put the vast health institutional capacity to test here.

CONCLUSION

Violent conflict is a veritable obstacle to inter-state cooperation in general and in health. The case of the conflict in the eastern provinces of the DRC is an excellent example to cite here. The conflict persists to date, and the Norwegian Refugee Council declared the situation in the Congo as the world's most neglected refugee crisis. Rwanda continues to be accused of supporting the pro-Tutsi militia named the M23. In this conflict, refugees and internally displaced people have paid a huge price. Because of a total breakdown in the health system, infectious diseases like Cholera and EVD have taken a devastating toll on the population especially refugees. The regions of the north and south Kivu are no strangers to deadly misery as it has witnessed the operation of over 120 militia groups that regularly rape, terrorise, and kill. It is also the site of the world's second-largest Ebola outbreak. With a breakdown in national security, health workers including humanitarian volunteers strive to help the sick by putting their own lives on the line as some villages are considered too dangerous for health workers to visit. Being a cauldron or crucible of multi-ethnic conflicts involving the Tutsi, Hutus, Batwa, Hunde, Nyanga and Nande tribes, as well as foreign interests in its mineral wealth notably from Uganda and Rwanda, international terrorism, inter-group distrust and even the suspicion of the intentions of humanitarian and health workers is rife. That some of them like the M23 and the ADF are proxies for foreign exploitation makes a negotiated settlement extremely difficult. President Felix Tshisekedi declared a state of siege in both North Kivu and Ituri and appointed military governors to pacify the regions, but the fighting has continued. In February 2022, 94 people were killed at a camp for IDPs in Djugu territory, and on March 29, 2022, eight UN soldiers died in an unexplained helicopter crash in North Kivu although Kinshasa blamed the pro-Tutsi M23 for the incident. Relations between Rwanda and the DRC are at an all-time low and although former Kenyan President Uhuru Kenyatta's suggestion for a regional military force to be deployed in eastern Congo has been accepted by President Felix Tshisekedi, he has vehemently ruled out the participation of Rwanda. The admission of the DRC into the EAC and the planned military intervention of peacekeeping troops from this community could be the beginning of a diplomatic and negotiated settlement to the crisis because it may expose and blunt the teeth of Rwanda in the region.

REFERENCES

Africa Center for Strategic Studies. (2021, March 9). *Autocracy and instability in Africa*. Africa Center for Strategic Studies. https://africacenter.org/spotlight/autocracy-and-instability-in-africa/.

Bates, R. H. (2008). *When things fell apart: State failure in late-century Africa*. Cambridge University Press. https://doi.org/10.1017/CBO9780511790713

BBC News. (2020, July 23). Nigeria's Boko Haram crisis: Aid workers 'killed' in Bornu State. https://www.bbc.co.uk/news/world-africa-53511389

Britannica, T. (2022, November 24). Léon M'ba. *Encyclopedia Britannica*. https://www.britannica.com/biography/Leon-Mba.

Deltombe, T., Domergue, M., & Tatsitsa, J. (2016). *La guerre du Cameroun: L'invention de la Françafrique*. La Découverte.

Ewang, A. (2019). *Insurgents in Nigeria hold six aid workers: Attack on relief agencies worsen humanitarian crisis*. Human Rights Watch. https://www.hrw.org/news/2019/07/25/insurgents-nigeria-hold-6-aid-workers

Fabricius, P. (2019, August 22). *Reality check: Africa's bid to silence the guns*. Institute for Security Studies, South Africa. Institute for Security Studies. https://issafrica.org/iss-today/reality-check-africas-bid-to-silence-the-guns.

Gully, P. R. (2020). Pandemics, regional outbreaks and sudden-onset disasters. *Health Care Management Forum, 33*(4), 164–169. https://doi.org/10.1177/0840470420901532

Hegre, H. (2000). Development and the liberal peace: What does it take to be a trading state? *Journal of Peace Research, 37*(1), 5–30. https://www.jstor.org/stable/425723

Hodgkin, T. (1956). Nationalism in colonial Africa. *Sudan Notes and Records,* *37*(1956), 126–130. https://www.jstor.org/stable/41716729

Ikome, F. N. (2012). *Africa's international borders as potential sources of conflict and future threats to peace and security.* Institute for Security Studies. https://www.files.ethz.ch/isn/145411/Paper_233.pdf.

Jacquemot, P. (2010). The dynamics of instability in eastern DRC. *Forced Migration Review, 36,* 6–7. https://www.fmreview.org/sites/fmr/files/FMRdownloads/en/DRCongo/06-07.pdf

Joseph, R. (1978). *Gaullist Africa: Cameroon under Ahmadu Ahidjo.* Fourth Dimension Publishers.

Kadir, A., Garcia, D. M., & Romero, F. (2019). New ways to measure the effects of armed conflict in civilian populations. *The Lancet, 7*(12), 1586–1586. https://doi.org/10.1016/S2214-109X(19)30452-8

Kajeguka, A. (2019, August 26). *East African Community regional contingency plan for epidemics due to communicable disease, conditions, and other events of public health concern 2018–2023.* EAC Regional Knowledge Management Portal For Health. https://health.eac.int/publications/eac-regional-contingency-plan-for-epidemics-2018-2023#gsc.tab=0.

Kalipeni, Z., & Oppong, J. (1998). The refugee crisis in Africa and implications for health and disease: A political ecology approach. *Social Science Medicine, 46*(12). https://doi.org/10.1016/s0277-9536(97)10129-0

Lawson, B. S., Kelly, K. T., Parker, M., Colloton, K., & Watkins, J. (2010). *Reconstruction under Fire: Case studies and further analysis of civil requirements.* RAND Corporation. https://www.rand.org/content/dam/rand/pubs/monographs/2010/RAND_MG870.1.sum.pdf.

Levy, B. S., & Sidel, V. W. (2016). Documenting the effects of armed conflict on population health. *Annual Review of Public Health, 37,* 205–218. https://doi.org/10.1146/annurev-publhealth-032315-021913

Loretti, A. (1997). Armed conflicts, health and health services in Africa. An epidemiological framework of reference. *Medicine, Conflict and Survival, 13*(3), 219–228. https://doi.org/10.1080/13623699708409342

Mengisteab, K. (2003). Africa's intrastate conflicts: Relevance and limitations of diplomacy. *African Issues, 32*(1–2), 25–39. https://doi.org/10.2307/1535098

Murray, C. L., King, G., Lopez, A. D., Tomijima, N., & Krug, E. G. (2002). Armed conflict as a public health problem. *British Medical Journal, 324*(7333), 346–349. https://doi.org/10.1136/Fbmj.324.7333.346

Njenga, F. G., Nguithi, A., & Kang'ethe, R. N. (2006). War and mental disorders in Africa. *World Psychiatry, 5*(1), 38–39. https://www.ncbi.nlm.nih.gov/pmc/articles/PMC1472262/#:~:text=The%20most%20commonly%20encountered%20mental,and%20somatization%20disorder%20at%2072.2%25

Reyntjens, F. (2022, June 14). *Here they come again: The troubled relations between Rwanda and the Congo.* Italian Institute for International Political Studies. https://www.ispionline.it/en/pubblicazione/here-they-come-again-troubled-relations-between-rwanda-and-congo-35415.

Ross, M. L. (2004). What do we know about natural resources and civil war? *Journal and Peace Research, 41*(3), 337–356. https://doi.org/10.1177/0022343304043773

Russo, J. (2022, December 12). *The east African community steps into the crisis in the DRC. Will it help?* IPI Global Observatory. https://theglobalobservatory.org/2022/12/east-african-community-crisis-drc/

Sato, R. (2019). Effect of armed conflict on vaccination: Evidence from the Boko haram insurgency in northeastern Nigeria. *Conflict and Health, 13*(49). https://doi.org/10.1186/s13031-019-0235-8

Siddique, A. K. (1994). Cholera epidemic among Rwandan refugees: Experience of ICDDR,B in Goma, Zaire. *Glimpse, 16*(5), 3–4. https://pubmed.ncbi.nlm.nih.gov/12288419/

Siegle, J. (2021, December 17). *Africa's coups and the role of external actors.* Africa Center for Strategic Studies. https://africacenter.org/spotlight/africas-coups-and-the-role-of-external-actors/.

Siegle, J., & Cook, C. (2020, September). *Circumvention of term limits weakens governance in Africa.* Africa Center for Strategic Studies. https://africacenter.org/spotlight/circumvention-of-term-limits-weakens-governance-in-africa/.

Smith, A. M., & Jeppesen, C. (2017). *Britain, France and the decolonisation of Africa: Future imperfect?* UCL Press. https://doi.org/10.2307/j.ctt1mtz521

United Nations. (n.d.). Migration dynamics, refugees, and internally displaced persons in Africa. https://www.un.org/en/academic-impact/migration-dynamics-refugees-and-internally-displaced-persons-africa

United Nations Security Council. (2020). Letter dated 23 December 2020 from the group of experts on the democratic Republic of the Congo addressed to the President of the Security Council. https://digitallibrary.un.org/record/3896010?ln=zh_CN.

UNOCHA. (2021). Democratic Republic of the Congo: Violence against health care in conflict 2021. https://reliefweb.int/report/democratic-republiccongo/democratic-republic-congo-violence-against-health-care-conflict-2021

Venugopalan, H. (2016). Understanding the conflict in Congo, ORF Issue Brief, No. 139. https://orfonline.org/wp-content/uploads/2016/05/ORF_IssueBrief_139_Venugopalan_Final.pdf.

Waterbury, M. A. (2020). Kin-State politics: Causes and consequences. *Nationalities Papers, 48*(5), 799–808. https://doi.org/10.1017/nps.2020.3

Crisis Communication in Twenty-First Century Diplomacy: Implications for Digital Transformation of Foreign Policy

Henry Ngenyam Bang

INTRODUCTION

Digitalization and globalization are shaping foreign policy with implications for international politics and diplomacy (Riordan, 2019). Theoretical and practical interest in digital diplomacy (DD) has been growing over the years, influenced by the desire to understand the application of technology in mitigating the growing political, social, economic, and health crises facing the world. DD has distorted traditional ways of carrying out foreign policy actions and is now perceived as the various means by which diplomacy interacts with digital technology (Bjola & Holmes, 2015). The notion that foresight and risk consciousness are central to diplomacy is now being challenged by digitalization which involves risk-taking and communicating with an unknown audience (Hedling & Bremberg, 2021).

H. N. Bang (✉)
Department of Disaster and Emergency Management,
Coventry University, Coventry, UK
e-mail: henry.bang@coventry.ac.uk

H. N. Ndi et al. (eds.), *Health Diplomacy in Africa*, Studies in
Diplomacy and International Relations,
https://doi.org/10.1007/978-3-031-41249-3_7

143

How crises are communicated is fundamental to effective crisis management, which has been shaped by digitalization over the past decades (Cheng, 2018). This has implications for how Ministries of Foreign Affairs (MFAs) now conduct crisis communication (CC) in foreign policy. For instance, communication plays a key role in health crises, especially global crises as evidenced by the COVID-19 pandemic when governments communicate domestically to their populace (Bang, 2021) and the authorities can also project their foreign policy regarding coronavirus management. Indeed, CC has been fundamental in fostering global health diplomacy (GHD), which has been credited as relevant to improve global health, advancing social equity/justice, improving natural security and the relationship between states, and fostering collective development (Alkhaldi et al., 2021; WHO, 2020).

How governments communicate crises has implications for their reputation internationally and influences how their citizens and the international community perceive the crises. Yet, CC paradigms in foreign policy and diplomacy have shifted over the past six decades, sculpted by forces of globalization and the increasing digitalization of the world (Gilsinan, 2020). In the past few decades, digital platforms have been instrumental in communicating various crises including those caused by natural hazard-induced disasters, technological, social and anthropogenic hazards, complex emergencies, wars, and/or civil conflicts. Indeed, social media spaces have been used to crowdsource aid, appeal to people/communities, condemn atrocities, and document human rights violations. Online platforms have also been used for negative purposes like spreading disinformation, recruiting terrorists, and inciting violence. This has been the case in African countries (FATF, 2018) plagued with civil wars like Libya and Ethiopia. Hence the complex nature of digital platforms as a tool for CC is increasingly being scrutinized and has been further interrogated in this chapter.

The chapter argues that the changing dynamics of CC, which is principally influenced by the digital revolution, have implications on how MFAs craft, articulate, disseminate, and implement CC messaging to a wider audience. This has had implications for the operational effectiveness of the diplomats' communicative capabilities in view of the increasing role that digital media plays in CC (Cassidy, 2018). Now facing heightened responsibilities to act as the vocal gatekeeper of their country's foreign policy, diplomats' roles have become more complex during crises. By carrying out their government's message, they act as messengers to facilitate achieving specific aims/objectives for desirable outcomes during a crisis. This was aptly demonstrated during the COVID-19 pandemic.

In times of international health crises like the coronavirus pandemic, MFAs are under pressure to come up with policies on time and to ensure any measures taken are supported with information that is appropriate and relevant to the unfolding crisis. This was the case during the COVID-19 pandemic. Communication as a strategic tool in crisis management was underscored during the pandemic, especially in Africa where the continents' governments made relentless efforts to communicate adopted infection control measures to their domestic populace and the international community (Bang, 2021). Nevertheless, the role played by online platforms to strengthen the CC needs scrutiny (Gilsinan, 2020) since prior to the pandemic DD in Africa was arguably still very limited.

African diplomacy had been functioning in the old paradigm with the dominant use of conventional channels of communication. Digital communication in Africa is relatively sparse, and underdeveloped and has been leveraged more for domestic communication than diplomatic purposes (Wekesa, 2020). Nevertheless, the increasing uptake of digital communication in the continent has been influencing DD and one could say that Africa has leapfrogged into the digital age of diplomacy following the COVID-19 pandemic. The continent now needs to strategically position itself and strengthen its outreach in DD.

Underpinned by the dominance of digital information and communication technology in this era, this chapter examines DD and foreign policy communicative ability/capacity during crises with a focus on Africa. How twenty-first-century technological advancements are influencing diplomatic communicative strategies is examined, particularly the use of DD and social media platforms. Primarily, the increasing role of digitalization on diplomatic CC is explored. The chapter contributes to the literature on our understanding of contemporary diplomatic CC with implications for operational CC in foreign policy. The key argument is underpinned by the thesis that digital diplomatic CC is now a strategic foreign policy tool that MFAs must embrace, albeit with caution.

Conceptual Clarity in Digital Diplomacy: Concise Underpinnings

Diplomatic Signalling (DS)

The phrase "*diplomatic signalling*" (DS) has become common parlance in the literature of diplomatic communication and is increasingly being used synonymously with diplomatic messages. Classic diplomatic communication is perceived as a system of signals, which could be verbal as well as non-verbal (Constantinou et al., 2016). This involves diplomatic language that enhances cross-cultural communication among members of the profession (Jönsson & Aggestam, 1999). Indeed, uncertainty and unforeseen incidents may cause unintended signalling when stakeholders interpret behaviours/attitudes differently. Therefore, DS occurs when actors display attitudes/behaviours that are perceived, interpreted, or understood by others, irrespective of the mode of communication (Danielson & Hedling, 2021). Cassidy (2018) assert that in diplomatic settings, signals (digital or not) are used to package diplomatic messages and can serve to contradict or reinforce messages. The transition from DS to digital diplomatic signalling (DDS) is essentially in the medium of communication.

Digital Diplomatic Signalling (DDS)

Digital diplomatic signalling (DDS) is conceptualized as a message carried out through a digital medium by diplomats/state officials—whether intended or not—as a symbolic representation of the state's position on a particular matter. It has influenced the evolution of the way MFAs and their diplomatic services abroad apply various communication tools to enhance their foreign policy objectives when there is a crisis. Five key components influence the process of DSS and how states design messages and exert their foreign policy reach digitally. These elements are the sender's status, structure/design of messages, frequency of messages, the content of messages, and recipient of messages. A more in-depth examination of these components is in the following sections.

Sender's Status

The person, official, status, or rank of the diplomat to whom the online message is accredited or who sends the online message is important. In

CC, senior government officials or those in charge of managing crises would communicate key issues regarding the crisis with the intent that it would reach the targeted population who are expecting guidance from the government. This could be done via spokespersons or heads of diplomatic missions or Ambassadors if the messages are intended for an international audience. Depending on the diplomatic mission or its communication policies, senders could range from junior to senior diplomats or Heads of Consular Services or Embassies (ambassadors) or their spokespersons. At the middle of the spectrum are middle-ranking officials in some instances. There is obviously a correlation between the status of the sender and the robustness or strength of the message sent.

The volume and/or complexity of the incident to be dealt with has implications for the bureaucratic CC hierarchy. In contemporary diplomatic CC, the most senior officials (Ministers or Ambassadors) may not be in the position to respond to all issues or make the final decision. Depending on the specific crisis issue, that decision may be in the hands of other government officials, lower down the hierarchy, hence a response from other officials, especially if the state involved has established specific lines of communication (Spence & Batora, 2015). The online presence of senior diplomatic staff projects some reputation or prestige of the state they represent as being versed in current affairs or a crisis issue that is unfolding. Regular online discourses addressing key crisis issues are seen to further foreign policy objectives and are commended in this age of ICT.

Structure/Design of Messages

How messages address their subject matter or how they are framed or designed is relevant for DDS. Message structure/design involves the arrangement of words, sounds, images, and motion with the main aim of effectively communicating meaning to specific audiences in a particular context (Bishop, 2015). Message structures can be informal or formal, with both serving different purposes. The choice of words and tone vary between the two. Informal structures are more spontaneous and casual while a formal structure has the desire to show respect without compromising professionalism (Brown & Lewis, 2022).

Past diplomatic communication was usually very formal, with well-styled messages intended for a particular purpose and audience. The structure and way the messages were framed reflected the status of the diplomat. In this age of digital media, messaging is less structured, shorter in length, and informal on social media platforms. Two clear structures of messaging (Direct and Indirect) are noticeable on giant social media platforms like Facebook and Twitter. Direct messages from officials in diplomatic institutions make a great impact on their recipients. The messaging could be between diplomatic peers/colleagues (online official-to-official communication between diplomatic agents of the same country or other countries), official messages from diplomatic missions to their citizenry or intended for the citizens of other countries.

Indirect messages are demonstrated, for instance, when diplomatic staff join certain groups on Facebook or use the platform to "like" some messages sent by others. Indirect messages can also be sent when diplomats use their Twitter accounts to retweet key information from other posts. These messages are of significance especially when diplomats or their services/countries decide to retweet or like information on Facebook on a regular basis. This reinforces the messages or crisis discourse indicating its significance to the populace. Indirect messages, however, are ambiguous because the intent of the officials is not clear.

Whether the diplomat wishes to engage in the issue or endorse the discourse is not clear by simply retweeting and/or "liking" messages on Twitter or Facebook. One can argue that "liking" messages or retweeting them mean endorsing or agreeing with the dialogue. Notwithstanding, Cassidy (2018) note that many diplomatic official accounts caution that retweeting messages does not necessarily means an endorsement of the messages. As mentioned earlier, this may be a strategy to maintain flexibility to disclaim signals if they, later, prove not to be popular with the population.

Frequency of Messages

The frequency of messages has been mentioned under indirect messages but warrants further discussion. Frequency is conceptualized as the amount of time the responsible foreign office official, or diplomat spends online, in the context of this chapter, during a crisis and what the audience receiving the messages perceive about the regularity of the messaging and the issues being addressed. This has relevance in DD since it arguably indicates the degree of relevance of the discourse that either warrants or does not warrant the time of the diplomat. Archetti (2010) carried out empirical research on the media impact on diplomatic practice with foreign diplomats in London and found that the frequency of exchanges between diplomats influenced the level of political interest towards a foreign country in the UK.

Online signalling is strong if the posting is frequent. The audience will feel that the issue or crisis being discussed is important and would view the diplomats or their institution as active in the discourse. This projects the image of active virtual engagement, relevant in this fast-paced era of online information dissemination. The reputation of the diplomatic service would be further enhanced if more diplomatic staff are perceived to be engaged in the online discussion of the crisis. Conversely, if the diplomats and/or their institution decide to be silent on an issue that the populace or their diplomatic peers expect them to discuss, the signal being sent out could indicate the issue or crisis is not important. As highlighted earlier, silence as a diplomatic tool could be ambiguous, but strategic at the same time to sustain flexibility to be able to deny association with some messages or to conceal vital information (Cassidy, 2018). The speed of messages, nevertheless, has implications on their accuracy and the process that some messages can go through before being approved for public consumption.

Content of Messages

In crisis situations, diplomats are expected to rapidly update their audience on the situation in real-time or expedite their response to key inquiries on a crisis. Nevertheless, engaging in real-time dialogue, dissemination or response can dilute the content of messages or cause errors in the intent of messages if the messages being crafted are not properly vetted. Therefore, balancing the need for rapid communication and the quality of the messages is challenging in online diplomatic communication. In most instances, the need to disseminate more accurate and properly thought-through messages that provide the desired signals takes precedence over the speed of messaging. Having more accurate and tailored messages is arguably a more sensible thing to do to minimize communication errors. Once messages with errors have been sent out, it becomes substantially difficult to retract or correct them. This is worst if instructional messages were involved, and courses of action had been taken by the public based on the messages. The time that is taken to assess official messages or speeches before they are made public warrants further conceptual or practical examination and is beyond the scope of this chapter.

Recipient of Messages or Audience

The message recipients or targeted audience form part of the online signalling equation. This is commonly referred to as social media followers. Having the right social media platforms also influences the type/number of social media followers one can have, so it is necessary to have a strong social media presence on the most popular platforms to get the right outcome in terms of disseminating messages. Tips to attract more social media audience/followers include the use of hashtags to make your posts more discoverable and enhance engagement, posting relevant and interesting content, and connecting with others with whom you have similar interests (Bryaton, 2022).

In the context of digital communication, the reach of the messages is normally those following the diplomat's account online. This includes their friends, the public, or other social media users who may intentionally or accidentally notice diplomatic online messages. These people would normally possess a social media account that is the same as that of a diplomat or country. Since the diplomats may have a dedicated audience following their online activities, the implication is that they should also be able to listen and respond to their followers. The communication should be two-way traffic, not just one-way from the diplomat to the audience. The relevance of engagement in foreign policy cannot be overemphasized—engaging or responding to the concerns of the public fosters foreign policy goals and has the capacity to strengthen public trust in government actions during crises (Bang et al., 2020). Indeed, social media has just reinforced the old-age tradition of foreign policy engagement with the public and other diplomatic services. The level or intensity of engagement has been amplified by online platforms requiring diplomats to upgrade their engagement skills to exert their influence online.

CRISIS COMMUNICATION

CC has been conceptualized in various ways albeit in a similar context. It has been viewed as disseminating information to the public to avoid and/or recover from a crisis including enhancement of reputation (Fearn-Banks (2010). According to Coombs and Halladay, cited in Bang (2021) CC can be conceptualized from a broad perspective of collecting, processing, and disseminating information necessary to address a crisis (p. 78). Reynolds and Quinn (2008) conceptualize CC as endeavours to inform the population to coerce them to make informed decisions within a short time that could save their lives and/or property. Generally, the CC discourse is within a context that seeks to explain the potency of activities during a crisis, how they are done, and any limitations or challenges encountered (Bang, 2021). The scope of crisis communication has broadened in the twenty-first century with its application in several disciplines, including communication strategies in public health and diplomacy as analysed in this chapter.

Digital Medium

The term digital medium refers to the various communication or media platforms that enable or use digital content/delivery or interactivity by any means and at the disposal of the public. It could be for personal or commercial use and the platform could use the internet, mobile/digital technology, computer, or other networks for distribution, communication/display including social media platforms like Twitter, Instagram, Facebook, Snapchat, YouTube, Flickr, Weibo, VK, Google, websites or blogs, and apps.

Some of these digital mediums are now used by MFAs and diplomats to achieve their CC objectives including public engagement and gathering and disseminating information. Of these platforms, Twitter and Facebook have been more integrated into the diplomatic CC strategies of many MFAs. The advantages of using these platforms include but are not limited to the fact that they serve as a direct communication gateway linking MFAs, their citizens worldwide, and the international community. They are also cheaper to use, allowing for expedited information transmission on foreign policy or in some instances, consular assistance. Furthermore, their generic application in the context of crises, disasters, or emergencies has been noted—they facilitate the tracking of disaster victims, the most affected areas, or locations of people needing the most help (Cheng, 2018). Despite its importance, the relatively sparse information and communication technology infrastructure in Africa is limiting many countries in the continent from achieving their full digital potential.

Communicating Crises in Twenty-First-Century Diplomacy

The Shifting Perception of Crises

With predicted increases in the intensity and frequency of climate change-induced disasters, the world is poised to experience increasing natural hazards, crises, disasters, calamities, emergencies, and/or risks (Bang & Burton, 2021). How these crises are perceived and communicated has implications for effective crisis response. In a globalizing world characterized by unprecedented technological advancements, there has been a paradigm shift from the view that disasters/crises were acts of God or caused by natural processes to which humans have little control, to one that recognizes the human influence on the consequences of the crises. Indeed, crises are an inescapable fact of life, and we should recognize that crises would always be part of humanity and need to be dealt with using human ingenuity.

The dynamics of modern crises are increasingly becoming complex, characterized by politics, interdependence, globalization, and digitalization. Hence the need to better understand the nuances of modern crises, and how they are being dealt with. One area requiring in-depth research is how diplomats who are assigned the task of crisis management communicate state policies effectively. But the landscape of diplomatic CC has been changing over the past decades, influenced principally by digital media with positive and negative consequences. A notable limitation is that the digitalized global information space has facilitated crisis occurrence through the interdependence of global society with crises now transcending traditional state borders. This has resulted in cross-border social disarticulation and facilitated breeding grounds for extremist organizations (Chong, 2007).

Furthermore, global information and communication technology has framed the way twenty-first-century CC is perceived. In this light, '*information*' has become the key '*commodity*' by which education levels, knowledge, skills, progress, wealth, development, and well-being are assessed (Cassidy, 2018). Therefore, knowledge acquisition and information are critical for success in a conscientious information world. This has implications for MFAs, diplomatic institutions, and foreign policy during crises. That is why it is relevant to recognize the critical role that information technology is playing to influence diplomatic crisis management and communicative practices.

DIGITAL DIPLOMACY (DD)

The phrase "DD" was introduced in the US diplomatic setting in the 1990s and associated with the concept of '*soft*' power for leveraging diplomatic communication (Nye & Owens, 1996). Hedling and Bremberg (2021) define DD as "*a broad term that refers to how the internet, digital tools, digital media, and the technology sector have influenced or even transformed diplomacy*" (p. 1596). As mentioned in Pipchenko and Moskalenko (2017), the US Institute of Peace defines DD, as "a *form of foreign policy which is associated with the use of global information and communication networks in international relations and covers the practice of interstate relations, the system of foreign policy decision-making, communication of diplomatic missions carried out by means of information and communication technologies*" (p. 17). According to Bjola and Holmes (2015), DD encompasses all the various ways in which digitalization interacts with diplomacy. They view DD as both a driver and a result of digitalization. It is inevitable that DD will continue to influence international politics, not least the role of digital CC in foreign policy and how states communicate crises to both their domestic and foreign audiences.

A retrospective examination of CC in diplomacy reveals that DD evolved through the 1990s when MFAs started adopting and leveraging digital technologies, including the use of emails as opposed to diplomatic cables. By the 2000s some MFAs started publishing weekly blogs and about a decade ago, MFAs started experimenting with virtual embassies (Teleanu & Kurbalija, 2022). This practice featured regularly in the CC strategies of diplomats, which included life and/or pre-recorded news broadcasts, State visits by senior government officials like Ministers, Collective Representations, or Demarches. In such circumstances, the structure and language of communication were usually formal and delivered by senior diplomats such as Ambassadors (Cassidy, 2018). This way of conducting diplomacy, however, has gradually been changing over the years and is now under the auspices of DD.

The change from DS to DDS has been remarkable. Indeed, DDS brings a novel communication ability to contemporary CC. In order words, DDS is a core means of "*virtual state enlargement*" (Cooper & Shaw, 2009) in this media era dominated by digitalization and its influence on contemporary diplomatic communication. This has broadened the range of communicative potentials at the disposal of diplomats, notably social media platforms, signalling an almost complete paradigm change on how crises shall be communicated in future.

With this novelty in CC, one can state that the days when diplomatic signals were limited to recorded broadcasts or visits by senior state civil servants are nearly over! Foreign policy stakeholders in Africa must now recognize that a modern-day diplomat's CC arsenal functions in an environment that is dominated by digital media and must be prepared to engage in the social media platform. Nevertheless, it is imperative that diplomatic messages that are being crafted should be accurate, clear, transparent, and open to provide reassurance to the populace. In this light, designing messages in an open and empathetic manner would help to galvanize public trust and any required action (Bang, 2021; Reynolds & Quinn, 2008; Sellnow & Sellnow, 2019).

Online Diplomatic Networks

Networking at the state level is not a new phenomenon. It has existed for centuries, with the need for gathering, analysing, sharing, and reporting information. For instance, information deciphered from cuneiform tablets that were written in ancient Egypt reveals the need for intelligence to protect and sustain the Asian empire (Jönson & Hall, 2003). Nowadays, social media has made diplomatic networks novel in the speed and reach of messages within cohorts of diplomats. The way diplomatic stakeholders perceive messages received, and how they analyse and respond to the messages determine the degree of influence that diplomats have in contemporary digital CC. Cassidy (2018) underscore diplomatic networking signalling as not just a means of information dissemination amongst the diplomatic corps, but also as a medium of shared diplomatic norms, values, and ideas.

In crisis situations, diplomats publicly sharing their views and manifesting public support for the ideas of one another helps to boost or reinforce some messages, enabling the audience to take them more seriously. Regular resharing or retweeting messages on Facebook and Twitter in diplomatic networks increases the reach potential of the message. Public support for the information is also enhanced and there is a greater potential for the public to act on any instructional messages. Consequently, the power of diplomatic networks cannot be ignored or undermined as a significant diplomatic communication tool. But as analysed later in this chapter, online diplomatic networking is still gaining pace in African diplomacy.

Media Platforms for DD

Digital media platforms are instrumental in sustaining DDS. Notably, internal and external forces have influenced the adoption of digital technology or platforms. An internal motive is when an MFA embraces digital technology to achieve specific foreign policy aims. An example is algorithms developed by Israel's MFA to mitigate hate speech on Facebook. External incidents like political uprisings around the world facilitated the adoption of social media by diplomatic services to engage with foreign citizens. This DDS is happening in real-time in an online interconnected world where messages are being transmitted instantaneously to millions of people worldwide (Bang, 2021), facilitated by social media platforms like YouTube, Twitter, Facebook, etc.

The most prominent social media mediums are Twitter and Facebook. These platforms have become very popular and integrated within contemporary diplomatic CC measures. For instance, Twitter, in this age of ICT, demonstrates an evolved, distinct, and new means of disseminating a country's foreign policy in less than 280 characters. Many countries and their diplomatic missions now have Twitter accounts. The application of this social media platform is novel in the sense that diplomatic CC can now be designed and framed in linguistically short and informal messages and easily dispersed to much larger segments of the populace including wider demographics.

Twitter has broad and targeted outreach capabilities unmatched by other media platforms. The prevalence and presence of Twitter's hashtag (#) allow users to 'tag' posts to the wider conversation, enabling messages to reach international audiences in seconds/minutes. Therefore, Twitter users can easily access messages by searching for hashtags to see related content, regardless of whether the users follow the accounts or not. By limiting messages to only 280 characters, Twitter encourages brevity and succinct messages or communication that gets 'straight to the point'.

Studies have demonstrated the critical role of social media platforms during the COVID-19 pandemic. Due to travel restrictions or indoor policies during the peak of the pandemic, many countries, their diplomats, and the public started attending virtual meetings via Zoom, Teams, and other online platforms as opposed to normal face-to-face meetings. Their Twitter platform was extensively used to disseminate information on the virus spread, measures taken by the authorities to fight the pandemic, the requirements of the populace, and the concerns and priorities of the most vulnerable. In disseminating information or policy about the virus, messages used the #coronavirus hashtag or #covid19 in tweets. This ensured the tweets appeared in the search results of those looking to see the top/latest tweets about the virus. (Alomari et al., 2021). It should be noted, however, that while social media practices can positively affect CC, they have also produced ambiguous signalling capable of plunging the populace into a vortex of social media misinformation.

Ambiguous Signalling in Digital Diplomacy

Ambiguous signalling may be a prelude to disaster, for instance, between aeroplane pilots and air traffic controllers. It could also jeopardize legal situations and improve the chances of one or more parties raising a successful challenge in court. That is why strenuous efforts are made to eschew ambiguity in legal practice. This is not necessarily the case in diplomacy. Deception, dishonesty, and duplicity is an ancient practice in diplomacy that has thrived to this day. Its roots can be traced to ancient Greece, specifically the ancient Greek God known as Hermes who was very mischievous, crafty, cunning, and associated with deception, and trickery (Cartwright, 2019). It is believed he transferred such attributes and traits to his representative and envoys and have since been linked to diplomacy (Frey & Frey, 1999). This aligns with the statement by an English diplomat (Sir Henry Wotton) who is quoted to have said in 1604 that *"An ambassador is an honest man sent to lie abroad for the commonwealth"*. Wotton is also said to have advised a British diplomat to *"Ever speak the truth; for, if you will do so, you shall never be believed, and 'twill put your adversaries to a loss in all their dispositions and undertakings"* (Bent, 1887).

Ambiguity in diplomatic communication is viewed to be constructive or beneficial. Arguably, the concept has been employed by diplomats to avoid embarrassment and distance themselves from messages that receive a negative response or are unpopular. Ambiguity has also been favourable to diplomatic signalling for the following reasons: to hide key information between parties; to make it possible to disclaim any messages sent, which gives room for later arguments; and to maintain flexibility. Jönson and Hall (2003) observed that in diplomatic settings, unintended attitudes could send messages through social media. This situation can arise when diplomats wish to fly a 'trial balloon' and if "...*they do not have the time to present a clear position of where they may stand on the issue at play, or the situation is rapidly changing leaving them to be wary of presenting publicly a strong position*" (Cassidy, 2018, p. 9).

Ambiguity often arises when dealing with multiple audiences. While unambiguous messaging may be desirable for some receivers of messages, it might be bad for others. For instance, trying to communicate to local, national, regional, and international audiences. This was the case at the peak of the coronavirus pandemic when the international community loved to hear messages on strict infection control measures while the local population, especially in developing countries hated such messages due to the socio-economic impact on their lives and livelihoods.

The ambiguity of diplomatic signals is also fuelled by the prevalence of non-verbal messages in communication between countries. Hand gestures, facial expressions, body language, tone of voice, and posture involved in non-verbal communication could send mixed signals to receivers of messages. A diplomat's cultural background or where the person fits in with social settings may also influence their non-verbal cues and skills (Taylor, 2021). Indeed, understanding non-verbal cues could pose problems when trying to decipher messages.

Nonetheless, Jervis (1976) notes that diplomats are more apt to provide true than false information since countries pay keen attention to diplomatic communications and there is a need for heightened caution, not least for fear of losing trust and reputation to both the domestic and international audience should deception fail. Therefore, balancing the equation between the impetus for clarity and ambiguity shall require that diplomats should be more careful in crafting their messages and or exert much effort in preparing for and explaining signals (ibid).

COVID-19's Influence on African Digital Diplomacy

The coronavirus-induced restrictions on movements and gatherings created an uptick in digital diplomacy worldwide albeit challenging to African international diplomacy. Prior to the COVID-19 pandemic, African diplomacy had access to digital communication mainly through the ubiquity of digitalization, which ensured that all and sundry had access to social media platforms. This enabled African diplomatic missions to have some presence on digital platforms, plagued with some challenges in digital communication. A perusal of the use of digital platforms by African MFAs and diplomatic missions reveals that their websites are either rarely updated or poorly developed, and their diplomatic activities on professional platforms (LinkedIn) and search engine platforms (Google, YouTube) are light. Furthermore, their messaging on social media platforms like Twitter and Facebook is either erratic or missing. Wekesa (2020) assets that digital communication in Africa has been leveraged more for domestic communication than diplomatic purposes.

Surveys on Twitter, Facebook, and Instagram reveal intermittent DD activity by some African leaders and diplomats (BCW, 2022), including the use of WhatsApp as a tool for CC. A good example was its use by South African diplomats in 2020 to respond to the xenophobic attacks on foreigners in South Africa amidst measures to curb the violence. Nevertheless, some analysts considered the use of basic digital platforms as an exception, rather than a rule since, for example, few African leaders like Paul Kagame (Rwanda), Nana Akufo-Addo (Ghana), and Uhuru Kenyatta (Kenya) used it regularly (Wekesa, 2020).

The coronavirus pandemic enhanced DD engagement of African MFAs. Previously, African diplomats may have attended teleconferences intermittently, but the pandemic left them no choice but to attend and communicate their crisis management strategies to peers online. As the health crisis unfolded, many African foreign ministers and presidents were forced to attend virtual bilateral/multilateral conferences/meetings. The presidents of the Economic Community of West African States (ECOWAS) held several video conferences to discuss solutions to the pandemic. Comparatively, it may be fair to argue that African countries were lagging in terms of DD and digital platforms were mundane in African diplomacy prior to the COVID-19 pandemic (ibid). Notwithstanding, the coronavirus pandemic showed that DD is becoming more firmly anchored in African foreign policy against a backdrop of gloomy predictions and dreaded scenarios, which did not materialize. Although limited prior to the pandemic, the unprecedented use of virtual conferencing in bilateral/multilateral video conferences to address the pandemic management shows that African countries can adapt fast to DD.

DD was also used to facilitate the exchange of information and best practices on COVID-19 response efforts. For example, the African Union (AU) launched a platform called the Africa COVID-19 Response portal which provided a central hub for sharing information and resources related to the pandemic. The organization also used social media to disseminate information on COVID-19 prevention and control measures, including to advocate international support for Africa's fight against the pandemic. In the heat of the crisis, the Chairperson of the African Union Commission, repeatedly twitted several messages requesting assistance from within Africa and Africa's diaspora communities to help the AU raise the sum of US$ 1 million for the AU COVID-19 Response Fund (@AUC_MoussaFaki, 25/05/2020 at 18:42). Similarly, addressing the Vaccine and Global Security Session of the G7 Foreign and development Ministerial meeting, Moussa Faki lamented through social media, the disproportionate delays, in comparison with the rest of the world, not only of the vaccines ordered on the market but also those pledged under the Covid-19 Vaccines Global Access (COVAX) facility. These messages are escalated at the levels of different AU Commissions, regional economic communities, foreign ministries, and ministries of public health. Whereas digital communication may be efficient in carrying the AU's views to its international partners and the global world of mass media, its effect on the African populace is limited. The reason is a limited internet network coverage in most countries that covers a relatively small geographical space, mostly in big towns/cities. The cost to access the networks is also relatively high and most of the populace cannot afford it. By far the commonest social media platform is WhatsApp, which is limited only to those a communicator has telephone contact with.

Though plagued with challenges, the African digital foreign policy scene is promising, and the continent's DD journey is on course and could be expedited if certain initiatives are taken. While it may be difficult to associate the coronavirus pandemic with any positives, there are opportunities that emerged from dealing with the challenges brought about by the pandemic. For instance, the limited use of ICT by African diplomats during the crisis is a challenge that needs examining as an opportunity for improving digital communication in African health diplomacy. Africa needs to improve its competencies in internet governance and DD to navigate CC in real time. This can be done by mobilizing human, financial, and institutional resources to advance their digital foreign policy objectives. That would ensure more prominence and active engagement of African foreign policy stakeholders on the global digital stage to advance their priorities, goals, and interest. I believe Africa's digital dynamism shall certainly grow as the continent continues to play an increasing role in international affairs via digital governance. Overall, digital diplomacy has been an important tool for African governments in their efforts to respond to the COVID-19 pandemic and coordinate with international partners.

Discussion and Conclusion

This chapter has conceptually examined digital CC in foreign policy. By examining how diplomats use CC in international politics, the chapter has underscored the relevance of online digital platforms in facilitating the process. Over the last century, perceptions of the causation, intensity, and impact/effects of crises have been shifting with increasing knowledge and understanding of vulnerability and resilience to natural hazards and political crises, including complex emergencies. This paradigm shift is influencing how governments manage both domestic and foreign crises, with CC now playing a pivotal role in crisis management. The chapter has underlined the power of online DS and how this communicative ability can foster foreign policy goals through real-time digital communication. It has emphasized that MFAs have now embraced digital media as an inevitable tool for CC.

The increasingly relevant role that social media plays in foreign policy and international politics has been underscored and the influence of key media platforms in aiding this digital transformation has been addressed. Facebook and Twitter platforms have been used as examples to show how DS influences foreign policy communication. The main characteristics of DDS have been highlighted, and the tools have been used to show how diplomats can effectively utilize them in an online communication strategy during a crisis.

While the positive impact of DD warrants to be praised, we should be cautious and critically examine the complex dynamics involved in the digital application of diplomacy. The issue with the use of digital media platforms is that it is not a level playing field. Some countries may be more proficient than others in using social media platforms to pursue their foreign policy aims and diplomats skilled in communication may use digital platforms to sway international public perceptions.

The ambiguity of messages on social media platforms can be perceived as a prominent way in which states can manipulate public opinion. When ambiguous messaging is used to influence public opinion, the public might be intentionally deceived. Social media messages like Tweets, videos, and images posted online have the potential to provide both positive and negative reactions with the potential of calming or inciting/

exacerbating crises. Consequently, state digital disinformation campaigns can wrongly sway public opinion in a situation of crisis, leading to the wrong reactions or noncompliance with instructional messaging. This is morally wrong albeit the states might achieve their foreign policy objectives in the short term. The risk with controversial or ambiguous messages as a foreign policy tool is that the public may demand further explanation or clarification if they doubt the authenticity and/or truthfulness of messages from diplomatic sources. Some states may decide to be quiet or not respond in such circumstances, but not being responsive to shifts in public opinion can impact public trust in diplomatic communication. That is why this chapter strongly advocates a 'two-way street' communication dynamic where diplomats are obliged to respond to queries from their messages. Since managing public opinion or reaction to messages posted online is difficult, MFAs should be cautious and avoid deceitful messages for the sake of short-term foreign policy gains. It would be a daunting prospect to contain the long-term often negative reactions if the disseminated messages are found to be intentionally misleading.

The fast-paced nature of contemporary communication, facilitated by digital technology, has invariably made it inevitable for countries, their MFAs, and individual diplomats to have no choice but engage with digital communication. The analysis shows that modern diplomacy is now conducted in a digital playfield requiring all countries to partake in the game, albeit African countries have challenges in the knowledge and/or effective use of digital technology. With digital tools becoming invaluable in conventional diplomacy, an overwhelming proportion of countries either have or are soliciting accounts on online media platforms especially popular ones like Twitter and Facebook. Embracing this novel online diplomacy has implications for the financial and human capital of African countries, whose diplomatic budgets are often much smaller compared to that of western countries. Based on this analogy, one can deduce that western countries would be more skilled in DD than those in the South.

Despite being relatively new, Africa's diplomatic system swiftly adjusted to the coronavirus pandemic with online conferences to discuss a variety of issues of regional and continental significance regarding the crises (Accord, 2020). Now that African MFAs have embraced DD, they need to put in place proper policies and strategies to leverage this novel practice since their urgent transition from physical to virtual meetings did not provide much time for planning. That should include the need for African diplomats to be formally trained/educated in DD. This can be led by

Research Institutes and Diplomatic Academies in African Universities. Indeed, the central objective of a conference on African Diplomatic Academies, Universities, and Research Institutes that was held in 2018 was to develop collaboration between Diplomatic Training and Research Institutes in the African continent (Kimble, 2018). One would of course expect DD policies to go beyond online conferences and encapsulate all aspects of digital foreign policy applications including CC. The DD policies would benefit African diplomacy in a variety of ways: facilitate greater investment to support fast/reliable internet connectivity; provide standardized digital communication; renew attention to cybersecurity; address the issues of inconsistencies, vagueness, or ambiguity in communication; aid diplomats to familiarize themselves with foreign policy objectives in line with African objectives; and advance digital economic development in Africa. Indeed, DD heralds a new era in diplomacy CC for Africa.

Based on the discourse in this chapter, one could argue that DD is real, is now a routine, and has come to stay in the African diplomatic system. Undoubtedly, future diplomacy will be characterized by wider information dissemination and a greater frequency of messages through social media platforms. The digital public space is also under constant political pressure with states using their political power to control public opinion by banning the dissemination of online information when it suits them. This action, arguably, is contrary to the widely publicized ethos of freedom of speech. Having recognized the power of social media platforms to shape their foreign policy and influence public opinion, most African countries will continue to engage their domestic and international audience through this online communication medium. Nevertheless, the effectiveness of social media platforms in building interpersonal trust between states and their citizens, and between diplomatic counterparts remains a subject for debate.

In summation, this chapter has illuminated how DDS is an invaluable CC tool that MFAs in Africa should inculcate into their governance strategy when dealing with crises and/or disasters. It contributes to the literature on diplomatic digital CC and provides guidance on DDS including practitioner use of this communication tool. How MFAs project state power warrants further research, both empirically and conceptually to further elucidate the ideas discussed in this chapter.

REFERENCES

Accord. (2020). *Africa's COVID-19 diplomacy reflects its commitment to multilateralism and collective action.* https://www.accord.org.za/analysis/africas-covid-19-diplomacy-reflects-its-commitment-to-multilateralism-and-collective-action/

AlKhaldi, A., Nigel, J., Chattu, V., Ahmed, S., Meghari, H., Kaiser, K., IJsselmuiden, C., & Tanner, M. (2021). Rethinking and strengthening Global Health diplomacy through triangulated nexus between policymakers, scientists, and the community in light of COVID-19 global crisis. *Global Health Research and Policy, 6*(12). https://doi.org/10.1186/s41256-021-00195-2

Alomari, E., Katib, I., Albeshri, A., & Mehmood, R. (2021). COVID-19: Detecting government pandemic measures and public concerns from twitter Arabic data using distributed machine learning. *International Journal of Environmental Research in Public Health, 8*(1), 282. https://doi.org/10.3390/ijerph18010282

Archetti, C. (2010, September 2–5). *Media impact on diplomatic practice: An evolutionary model of change.* Paper presented at the American Political Science Association (APSA) Annual Convention. https://usir.salford.ac.uk/id/eprint/12444/1/Archetti._Media_Impact_on_Diplomatic_Practice._An_Evolutionary_Model_of_Change.pdf

Bang, H., & Burton, C. (2021). Contemporary flood risk perception in England: Implications for flood risk management foresight. *Climate Risk Management, 32.* https://doi.org/10.1016/j.crm.2021.100317

Bang, H., Mbah, M., Ndi, H., Ndzo, J., Bang, H., Mbah, M., Ndi, H., & Ndzo, J. (2020). Gauging Cameroon's resilience to the COVID-19 pandemic: Implications for enduring a novel health crisis. *Transforming Government: People, Process and Policy., 15*(4), 658–674. https://doi.org/10.1108/TG-08-2020-0196

Bang, H. N. (2021). Applying the novel IDEA model for instructional health risk and crisis communication to explore the effectiveness of the COVID-19 crisis communication in Cameroon. *Journal of Emergency Management,* Special Issue on COVID-19, 20(7), 77–102. https://doi.org/10.5055/jem.0648

BCW. (2022). *Welcome to twiplomac.* https://www.twiplomacy.com/

Bent, S. A. (1887). Familiar short saying of great men. *Bibliogaphic Record.* https://www.bartleby.com/344/411.html.

Bishop, M. J. (2015). Message design for digital media. In J. M. Spector (Ed.), *Encyclopedia of educational technology* (pp. 502–504). Sage Publishing.

Bjola, C., & Holmes, M. (2015). *Digital diplomacy theory and practice.* Routledge.

Brown, L., & Lewis, K. (2022). The elementary forms of digital communication. *PLoS One, 17*(9), e0273726. https://doi.org/10.1371/journal.pone.0273726

Bryaton, D. (2022). *5 tips to attract more social media followers.* https://speed-ysense.com/attract-more-social-media-followers/

Cartwright, M. (2019). *Hermes, World History Encyclopaedia.* https://www.worldhistory.org/Hermes/

Cassidy, J. (2018). *Digital diplomatic crisis communication: Reconceptualising diplomatic signalling in an age of real-time governance.* Working Paper No 3. Oxford Digital Diplomacy Research Group. http://www.qeh.ox.ac.uk/sites/www.odid.ox.ac.uk/files/DigDiploROxWP3.pdf

Cheng, Y. (2018). How social media is changing crisis communication strategies: Evidence from the updated literature. *Journal of Contingencies and Crisis Management, 26,* 58–68. https://doi.org/10.1111/1468-5973.12130

Chong, A. (2007). *Foreign policy in global information space: Actualizing soft power.* Palgrave Macmillan.

Constantinou, C., Kerr, P., & Sharp, P. (2016). *The SAGE handbook of diplomacy.* SAGE Publications. https://doi.org/10.4135/9781473957930

Cooper, A. F., & Shaw, T. M. (2009). *The diplomacies of small states: Between vulnerability and resilience.* Palgrave Macmillan.

Danielson, A., & Hedling, E. (2021). Visual diplomacy in virtual summitry: Status signalling during the coronavirus crisis. *Review of International Studies., 19,* 1–19. https://doi.org/10.1017/S0260210521000607

FATF. (2018). *Financing of recruitment for terrorist purposes.* FATF Report. https://www.fatf-gafi.org/media/fatf/documents/reports/financing-recruitment-for-terrorism.pdf

Fearn-Banks, K. (2010). *Crisis communications: A casebook approach.* Lawrence Erlbaum Associates.

Frey, L. S., & Frey, M. L. (1999). *The history of diplomatic immunity.* Ohio State University.

Gilsinan, K. (2020). *How China is planning to win back the world.* https://www.theatlantic.com/politics/archive/2020/05/china-disinformation-propaganda-united-states-xi-jinping/612085/

Hedling, E., & Bremberg, N. (2021). Practice approach to the digital transformations of diplomacy: Toward a new research agenda. *International Studies Review, 23,* 1595–1618. https://doi.org/10.1093/isr/viab027

Jervis, R. (1976). *Perception and misperception in international politics.* Princeton University Press.

Jönson, C., & Hall, M. (2003). Communication: An essential aspect of diplomacy. *International Studies Perspectives, 4*(2), 195–210. https://doi.org/10.1111/1528-3577.402009

Jönsson, C., & Aggestam, K. (1999). Trends in diplomatic signalling. In J. Melissen (Ed.), *Innovation in diplomatic practice. Studies in diplomacy.* Palgrave Macmillan. https://doi.org/10.1007/978-1-349-27270-9_9

Kimble, M. (2018). *Conference on African diplomatic academies.* Universities and Research Institutes. https://www.accord.org.za/news/conference-on-african-diplomatic-academies-universities-and-research-institutes/

Nye, J., & Owens, W. (1996). America's information edge. *Foreign Affairs.* https://www.foreignaffairs.com/articles/united-states/1996-03-01/americas-information-edge

Pipchenko, N., & Moskalenko, T. (2017). Trends of Ukraine's digital diplomacy. *European Political and Law Discourse, 4*(3). https://eppd13.cz/wp-content/uploads/2017/2017-4-3/04.pdf

Reynolds, B., & Quinn, S. (2008). Effective communication during an influenza pandemic: The value of using a crisis and emergency risk communication framework. *Health Promotion and Practice, 9*(4), 13–17. https://doi.org/10.1177/1524839908325267

Riordan, S. (2019). *Cyber diplomacy: Managing security and governance online.* Polity Press.

Sellnow, D., & Sellnow, T. (2019). The IDEA model for effective instrumental risk and crisis communication by emergency managers and other key spokespersons. *Journal of Emergency Management, 17*(1), 67. https://doi.org/10.5055/jem.2019.0399

Spence, D., & Batora, J. (2015). *The European external action service: European diplomacy post-Westphalia.* Palgrave Macmillan.

Taylor, P. (2021). *Nonverbal communication with examples.* https://bodylanguagematters.com/nonverbal-communication-with-examples/

Teleanu, S., & Kurbalija, J. (2022). *Stronger digital voices from Africa. Building African digital foreign policy and diplomacy.* https://www.diplomacy.edu/wp-content/uploads/2022/11/ENG_African-digital-foreign-policy_PUBLIC-report_WEB.pdf

Wekesa, B. (2020). *Covid-19 heralds the era of digital diplomacy in Africa.* https://uscpublicdiplomacy.org/blog/covid-19-heralds-era-digital-diplomacy-africa

WHO. (2020). *WHO foundation established to support critical global health needs.* https://www.who.int/news/item/27-05-2020-who-foundation-established-to-support-critical-global-health-needs

CHAPTER 8

Health in Climate Change Diplomacy in Africa

Estherine Lisinge-Fotabong

INTRODUCTION

Climate change has emerged in the last three decades as the most significant threat to sustainable development, especially in developing and low-income countries. The most conservative estimates indicate that the phenomenon presents the single biggest health threat facing humanity and is expected to cause approximately 250,000 additional deaths per year due to malnutrition, malaria, diarrhoea, and heat stress (WHO, 2021). Sustaining a healthy population requires access to clean air, safe water, and an adequate food supply and which is anchored on a stable climate conducive to human health and productivity.

The linkages between climate change and health have become more pronounced in recent years with the scientific analysis by the Intergovernmental Panel on Climate Change (IPCC), the United Nations body responsible for advancing knowledge on human-induced climate

E. Lisinge-Fotabong (✉)
African Union Development Agency (AUDA-NEPAD),
Johannesburg, South Africa

© The Author(s), under exclusive license to Springer Nature   167
Switzerland AG 2023
H. N. Ndi et al. (eds.), *Health Diplomacy in Africa*, Studies in
Diplomacy and International Relations,
https://doi.org/10.1007/978-3-031-41249-3_8

change paints an even grimmer picture of the impact of climate change on the health and well-being of populations around the world, especially those in poor and climate vulnerable communities in the global south. The Panel's recent 6th Assessment Report concludes that to prevent catastrophic health impacts and prevent millions of climate change-related deaths significant and coordinated actions are needed in climate-vulnerable countries, particularly in Africa (Adams et al., 2022). Following its nineteenth session held in Warsaw from 11–23 November 2013, the UN Framework Convention on Climate Change (UNFCCC) indicates that the impacts of climate change on health are very well documented and becoming widespread with heat-related mortality and increased disease transmission as direct consequences (UNFCCC, 2014). Similarly, the outcome document of the 3rd Africa Ministerial Conference on Health and the Environment held in 2018 also recognized the threats posed by climate change to human health and well-being (WHO & UNDP, 2018). The conference also highlighted the disproportionate impact of climate change on Africa due to existing vulnerabilities that have been precipitated by social, political, environmental, and economic conditions. Well-known vulnerabilities make African societies and economies highly exposed to the COVID-19 pandemic and its consequences (OECD, 2020). Some of these weaknesses are of particular concern. On the one hand, poor quality of healthcare, coverage and access, availability of medical personnel, especially in remote areas, and the prevalence of other diseases raise concerns about the response capacity on the health front.

For example, the rise in average temperature expands the environmental range of tolerance of a disease vector like the mosquito which causes malaria. Furthermore, desertification and soil deterioration will accelerate the loss of agricultural productivity, increasing malnutrition and associated ailments.

The climate crisis could erase substantial progress attained in the last half century in global health and poverty reduction, particularly for the poor, marginalized, and vulnerable populations. The phenomenon will potentially affect the attainment of Sustainable Development Goal 3 on ensuring healthy lives and promoting well-being for all. It increases the barriers to access and provision of good health care.

IMPACT OF CLIMATE CHANGE ON AFRICA'S HEALTH SYSTEMS

Climate change is likely to erase the progress and advances made by many African countries in the past fifty years in health and poverty reduction thereby jeopardizing the efforts at attaining universal health coverage. According to the World Bank, sub-Saharan which has the lowest Gross Domestic Product (GDP) per capita of US$1645 of any region of the world will be impacted significantly by climate change and will have a negative effect on the region's growth prospects (Hoogeveen & Lopez-Acevedo, 2021). Africa is heavily reliant on its natural and biodiversity resources for socioeconomic development and sustenance, and these are likely to be impacted by climate change with the loss of healthy life years predicted to be up to 500 times greater than in Europe. The continent which is historically the least contributor to climate change will be the most affected by negative impacts caused by rising temperatures, air quality, water supply safety, extreme weather event frequency and the quality of agricultural lands for food security and nutrition.

There is growing evidence about the impact of temperature rise and precipitation on cholera outbreaks in many parts of Africa with temperature rise driving epidemics and precipitation acting as a dispersal mechanism. For instance, in the 'State of the Climate in Africa' Report 2021, by the World Meteorological Organization, a cholera outbreak declared in Niger and Nigeria in 2021 was attributed to climate change. The report further states that the outbreak resulted from flooding and was compounded by inadequate waste management, poor sanitary and sanitation practices, lack of drainage systems, and consumption of contaminated water. The outbreak claimed the lives of 3300 people and affected almost 100,000 people mostly between the ages of 5 and 14 years (Ibid). Undoubtedly, climate change will have direct health implications for many populations with drivers such as extreme weather events likely to lead to increased levels of mortality and morbidity and changes in disease prevalence. The Africa Regional Office (ARO) of the World Health Organization (WHO) estimates that between 2001 and 2021, 56 percent of the public health events recorded in the African Region were climate related. Increases in temperature caused by climate change will result in ailments such as thermal stress, skin cancer, and eye diseases. Some cardio-respiratory diseases and allergic disorders are also attributable to a reduction in air quality arising out of climate change. However, according to the

World Health Organization, most of the health impacts of climate change are indirect with the manifestations mainly being malnutrition, neglected tropical diseases, diarrhoea, malaria, and meningitis amongst others.

AFRICA WITHIN THE CLIMATE CHANGE NEGOTIATIONS

International cooperation is important to achieve significant emission reductions for several reasons. First, climate protection is a public good that requires collective action, Second, international cooperation allows for linkages across policies at different scales, notably through harmonizing national and regional policies, as well as linkages across issues.

Africa is an important player in the global climate change negotiations and has championed many decisions at global fora on climate change and environmental sustainability. Key amongst the decisions achieved through the instrumentality of Africa is the principle of Common but Differentiated Responsibilities and Respective Capacities (CBDR-RC), which acknowledges the different capabilities and differing responsibilities of individual countries in addressing climate change, especially within the context of historical responsibilities. Africa has also been one of the most vocals in articulating enhanced actions on adaptation and climate financing. Africa has been active and visible right from the start of climate change negotiations. Notable structures in its participation include the Africa Group of Negotiators established since COP1 in Berlin, in 1995, forming the basis of a collective continental approach in the UNFCCC processes.

Africa's engagement within the global climate change discourse has been structured through a three-tier arrangement led by the Committee of African Heads of State on Climate Change (CAHOSSC). The Committee, which is a sub-component of the African Union (AU) Assembly, was established in 2009 by the 13th AU Assembly of Heads of State and Government ahead of the Copenhagen COP 15 is at the top of the decision-making process and provides high-level leadership and advocacy for an African Common Position on Climate Change and ensures that Africa speaks with one voice in the global climate change negotiations. The Committee has a membership of twelve Heads of States representatives of the regional blocs of the African Union. It seats during the Statutory meetings of the AU as well as during COP meetings. Its agenda includes receiving updates from the African Group of Negotiators and the African Ministers Conference on Environment (AMCEN) on Climate Change Initiatives and deliberations on the outcomes of global climate summit (COP) meetings and the implications for Africa. Its decisions are presented to the AU assembly for adaptation by the committee of the whole, which becomes the African Common Position.

The African Ministerial Conference on Environment (AMCEN) established in 1985 has become the main policy and agenda setting for environmental issues on the continent. The body is made up of African Ministers responsible for the environmental portfolio and is the main forum for discussing all environmental issues and initiatives of relevance to Africa with issues of climate change a permanent feature on the agenda of AMCEN.

The third component of the climate change negotiating architecture is the African Group of Negotiators on Climate Change, which is the technical body that engages in the technical components of the negotiations. The AGN prepares and drafts the text and common positions, guided by decisions and key messages from CAHOSCC and AMCEN. It is composed of negotiators from all AU member states and was established since COP1 in Berlin, in 1995 forming the basis of a collective continental approach in the UNFCCC processes. Though a key structure in the development of Africa's position in the UNFCCC process, support for its work is largely funded by partners (African Group of Negotiators on Climate Change, 2011).

In addition to the three structures discussed above, the African pavilion established at COP17 launched in Durban, South Africa, is a key platform and space hosted by the African Union Commission (AUC), African Union Development Agency (AUDA-NEPAD), African Development Bank (AFDB), and UNECA during COP meetings for hosting of African stakeholders to showcase Africa's best practices and successes in dealing with climate change and climate variability. The African Day is a high-level forum on Africa's future in the context of climate change. Africa's large presence in the least developed countries (LDC) block demonstrates robust negotiations and representation but also the value of Africa helping to raise and shape climate change debates (AfDB, 2022).

HEALTH DIPLOMACY WITHIN THE CLIMATE CHANGE NEGOTIATIONS

Health considerations within the global climate change negotiations have been given impetus as a key thematic area of the Nairobi Work Programme (NWP) on the impacts, vulnerability, and adaptation to climate change within the architecture of the UNFCCC (UNFCCC, 2014). The NWP is focused on making informed decisions on adaptation actions and measures that respond to climate change backed by sound scientific and socio-economic considerations. Africa through its Group of Negotiators makes submissions under the UNFCCC's Subsidiary Body on Scientific and Technological Advice (SBSTA) on the impact of climate change on human health including changes in the geographical distribution of diseases, and new and emerging health issues. Africa's submissions also highlight the impact of climate change as a driver of malnutrition, waterborne diseases, vector-borne diseases, and disaster impacts.

The African Union and its organs including the African Union Commission and the African Union Development Agency amongst others have pursued common African health diplomacy through diverse but complementary channels including multilateral platforms such as the United Nations and bilateral relationships. Significant progress has been made and international cooperation in health diplomacy deepened since 1926 when the first African medical interchange was held in West Africa. The conference brought together high-ranking colonial medical officers from some African countries alongside their counterparts from Britain, France, Belgium, Spain, and Portugal under the auspices of the League of Nations Health Organization (LNHO). The setup of the World Health Organization's Regional Office for Africa in 1952, in Brazzaville, the capital of the Republic of Congo represented a landmark moment in health diplomacy in Africa with the office being the first permanent regional organization exclusively focused on health in the region.

In the past decade, global health diplomacy has emerged as a new area of diplomacy between Africa and its partners in the global north and south. There have been some significant shifts within the context of donor-recipient relationships with Africa not just seen as a beneficiary of the largesse of the developed world but also playing an important role in finding innovative solutions to global health emergencies. Global health has opened a new frontier in development cooperation and diplomacy by adding another layer because it extends into previously unexplored spaces with diverse actors and diverse forms of negotiations.

For Africa, health diplomacy has assumed greater importance with the outbreak in 2014 of the deadly Ebola virus disease which claimed lives and ravaged the economies of some countries in the West Africa region. The AU response to Ebola started in April 2014 at the First African Ministers of Health Meeting jointly convened by the AUC and the WHO in Luanda, Angola (AU and WHO, 2014). A strong Communiqué and an appeal to Member States with experience in handling Ebola disease to assist were issued. The response was positive. Some AU Member States sent experts to the affected countries. $1,000,000 was released from the Union's Special Emergency Assistance Fund for Drought and Famine in Africa in August 2014 to finance response activities. The staff of the African Union also donated $100,000 to the collective Ebola response efforts (AU, 2015a). Global health diplomacy and cooperation were further tested with the onset of the COVID-19 pandemic that brought the world to a standstill. Vaccine nationalization and unequal access to vaccines exposed the chasm in global solidarity and breakdown in health diplomacy at both multilateral and bilateral levels. Despite these setbacks, global cooperation on health has improved significantly through engagements at different levels including 'mainstream diplomacy' with inter-country negotiations that happen largely within the United Nations architecture under the World Health Organization. For Africa, engagements under the African Union system have also become vigorous due to the growing interest and recognition of the critical role of robust health systems in national development. AU's response to the COVID-19 pandemic included the establishment of The African Union COVID-19 Response Fund which raised resources to strengthen the continental response to COVID-19. The fund supports pool procurement of diagnostics and other medical commodities for distribution to the Member States and the deployment of community workers and community healthcare workers to support contact tracing and mitigating the pandemic's socio-economic and humanitarian impact on African populations.

The creation of the Africa CDC as a continental public health institute to support member states' response to public health emergencies across the continent has boosted cooperation among African countries on health matters. The CDC has been at the forefront of catalysing cooperation and action in response to the COVID-19 pandemic.

COVID-19 demonstrated the inter-connectedness and transboundary nature of health challenges, and like climate change, they require robust negotiation, diplomatic, and cooperation systems. Multi-stakeholder health diplomacy where various bilateral and multilateral organisations work closely with national governments on national and regional health initiatives has proved increasingly relevant. In the past few years, many philanthropic organizations such as the Bill and Melinda Gates Foundation, the Welcome Trust, and the Pasteur Institute have played critical roles in health delivery in Africa, through their contribution of funding and scientific expertise in support of the goals for change in health and development.

Africa is a keen advocate of health diplomacy which is embedded in Aspiration one of Africa's Agenda 2063, the blueprint and vision for Africa's socio-economic development. The vision aims to build a prosperous Africa based on inclusive growth and sustainable development and work with a range of partners and coalitions for sustainable growth and development on the continent. Access to quality healthcare services for all people through investments in the health system is a key ambition of the vision (AU, 2015b).

Policies and initiatives at the level of the African Union have been adopted to address the nexus between health and climate change in Africa. The African Union has adopted a continent-wide strategy and action plan on climate change which acknowledges that climate change may negatively affect human health through the modification of the transmission of diseases such as cholera, malaria, meningitis, and zoonoses such as Ebola and the COVID-19 Coronavirus. The strategy estimates that the death rate from climate change is between 60 per cent and 80 per cent higher in Africa than in the next most vulnerable region (Southeast Asia) due to pre-existing vulnerabilities and weakened adaptation capacity. The strategy calls for the mainstreaming of climate change literacy into targeted sectors including health and encourages cross-sectoral approaches to adaptation planning that emphasize reducing risk across the climate change and health nexus (AU, 2022).

In 2003, the African Union under the guidance of the AMCEN adopted the Environment Action Plan of NEPAD as the first-ever continental Plan on environmental management in Africa. The Plan recognized the strong linkages between health and the environment and emphasizes the importance of integrating environmental considerations into poverty reduction policies and strategies including health systems across Africa (AU and NEPAD, 2003).

As a response to the Coronavirus pandemic, the Africa Union also adopted the Green Recovery Action Plan (July 2021), which recognizes that a clean and resilient recovery will create employment opportunities for the future whilst ensuring that the relationship between public health and climate change is addressed (AU, 2021).

In 2008, the Libreville Declaration on Health and Environment in Africa was adopted by a joint ministerial session of ministers responsible for health and the environment signed by 52 countries. The declaration aims at securing a political commitment from African governments towards strengthening the policy and institutional structures that will unlock investments to tackle environmental threats to health. Ten years on, the 3rd Inter-Ministerial Conference on Health and Environment in Africa adopted the Strategic Action Plan to scale up Health and Environment Interventions in Africa which aims at preserving ecosystem integrity and promoting healthy lives and well-being for Africans (WHO & UNEP, 2008).

Critical to addressing the linkages and nexus between climate change and health are the actions taken at the national level by member states and other stakeholders through nationally determined contributions (NDCs). The NDCs embody efforts by each country to reduce national emissions and adapt to the impacts of climate change with an ambition that is compatible with economic and social development. In terms of adaptation priorities, the 2021 NDC Synthesis Report, illustrate that Parties including African countries continue to focus on food production and nutrition security; freshwater resources; terrestrial and wetland ecosystems; human health; key economic sectors and services; disaster risk management and early warning; human habitats and urban areas; coastal areas and sea level rise; ocean ecosystems; and livelihoods and poverty. Almost all Parties outlined domestic mitigation measures as key instruments for achieving mitigation targets of their NDCs and/or targets for sectors or areas, such as energy supply, transport, buildings, industry, agriculture, and waste (UNFCCC, 2022).

The inclusion of health priorities in NDCs allows African countries to invest in climate-resilient and sustainable health systems. African institutions including AUDA-NEPAD provide capacity building and technical support to member states in this regard. The AUDA-NEPAD Climate Adaptation and Resilience Centre provides practical training to enhance knowledge of available global funding mechanisms for climate resilience building and skills to access these funds. For example, developing skills in coordinating the activities of major funds at the national level, e.g., Green Climate Fund (GCF) and Global Environment Facility (GEF), and in framing proposals with member states' NDC targets that deliver improved climate resilience at the local levels. It trains research leaders and policy-makers in the synthesis of evidence from climate information and other data across different sectors such as disaster, water, agriculture, health, and energy.

While considerable effort has been made to mainstream health in the climate change negotiations and related instruments such as the pro-gramme of work and the NDCs, much must be done about strengthening the voice of health professionals as advocates for stronger ambition on climate change in the UNFCCC process and national platforms in a scale like other sectors such as Agriculture and Food systems. It also must be acknowledged that there is a significant gap in facilitating access to climate change funding for health from the global climate change financings mechanisms such as GEF, Green Climate Fund, Adaptation Fund, and the GCF readiness programme.

The African Union system led by its member states and supported by its policy organs is committed to ensuring that the linkages between cli-mate change and health are addressed holistically given the increasing occurrences of health-related epidemics. Climate change and health diplo-macy as emerging areas are likely to become a central theme in addressing the hydra-headed challenges that face many countries, especially in Africa.

Despite these commitments in policy formulation and agenda setting, there is no gainsaying that Africa's health system needs a radical transfor-mation and investments to position it to respond to the emerging and anticipated impacts of climate change on human health and productivity. This would require a systemic design and shift by incorporating climate change considerations as a key component of public and primary health care at national and continental levels. This can be achieved by tackling the pervasive and extensive health inequalities in many parts of the continent that disproportionately affects the poor and marginalized in society.

Making an explicit link between health and climate change through the NDCs and sectoral plans, policies, regulations, and investment pro-grammes is central to the development of Health in Climate Change Diplomacy. Further inquiry into the practice, process, and tools needed to build climate-resilient and sustainable health systems as well as strengthen investment flow in adaptation and resilience is necessary. So too is the need to provide support to African member states in conducting research, developing, and promoting partnerships at all levels and across sectors and lastly securing financing to implement both adaptation and mitigation commitments and actions that have a positive impact on people's health.

CONCLUSION

In conclusion, health diplomacy has become critically important for global security and same as the defining roles of national governments, regional organisations, and non-state actors in fostering health cooperation in climate change diplomacy. Climate change is a public health issue, and the health sector has the ethical imperative of bolstering ambitious climate action. In the context of global climate diplomacy, countries must address trans-border issues that threaten global stability, including pandemics and climate change. Securing public health and well-being underscores all other forms of socio-economic development, and a healthy population is an asset to any nation. Therefore, it compels the pooling of resources and action at all levels and renewed forms of leadership that diplomatic efforts (through the AU) can help facilitate.

Regional organisations can effectively promote regional health diplomacy and governance through engagement with regional and global processes and frameworks. The Africa Union and its continental agencies and organs in recent times have played an important role in global climate change diplomacy as well as the development of regional health diplomacy and governance through the coordination of AU member states' participation in the UNFCCC negotiations and engagement in global negotiations with One voice in the Common African Position. The setting up of structures for Africa's participation in the UNFCCC process ensures coordination and an active contribution to the substantive issues on the agenda including the health and climate change linkages.

This role is primarily played by donors partnered with national governments. There is, however, a strong case to make for the more active involvement of regional economic communities (RECs) in health diplomacy and governance. For instance, in SADC, its capacity as a regional organisation, its role in the creation of social policy, the presence of member states and member state funding, and its relationship with donors and multilateral organisations in the region have been significant but can be strengthened further.

The gaps identified in the current literature include a lack of information on what the RECs do to advance regional health diplomacy and governance. The RECs can play a stronger role in facilitating and coordinating health governance and diplomacy through climate, environmental, and social policies, based on the potential capacity it has as a regional organisation.

For AU member states, taking an active role in mitigating climate change and adapting to its already inevitable impacts is imperative. The many co-benefits of climate action are particularly evident in health. For example, reducing air pollution has a direct impact on the prevention of diseases and premature death. WHO estimates that over a million lives could be saved every year by 2050 if air quality measures are implemented under the Paris Agreement. Such measures will necessitate a coordinated approach for focused health initiatives; political commitment including budgetary allocation of resources for adaptation and mitigation actions to implement the NDCs; and form partnerships at all levels to address systemic challenges of health systems, pervasive health inequalities which threaten the progress, and impact of health diplomacy at the national and continental level.

REFERENCES

Adams, H., Aldunce, P., Bowen, K., Campbell-Lendrum, D., Ebi, K., Hess, J., Huang, C., Liu, O., McGregor, G., Semenza, J., & Tirado, M. (2022). Heath, wellbeing and the changing structure of communities. https://www.ipcc.ch/report/ar6/wg2/downloads/report/IPCC_AR6_WGII_Chapter07.pdf

AfDB. (2022). Africa Pavilion. Africa Pavillon. https://www.afdb.org/en/cop27/africa-pavilion

African Group of Negotiators on Climate Change. (2011). https://africangroupofnegotiators.org

AU. (2015a). Africa Union: Fact sheet: Support to Ebola outbreak in West Africa. African Union and ASEOWA. https://au.int/sites/default/files/newsevents/workingdocuments/27015-wd-fact_sheet_1.pdf

AU. (2015b, September). Agenda 2063: The Africa we want. African Union Commission. https://au.int/sites/default/files/documents/36204-doc-agenda2063_popular_version_en.pdf

AU. (2021). African Union green recovery action plan 2021–2027. https://au.int/sites/default/files/documents/40790-doc-AU_Green_Recovery_Action_Plan_ENGLISH1.pdf

AU. (2022). African Union climate change and resilient development strategy and action plan (2022–2032). African Union. https://au.int/sites/default/files/

documents/42276-doc-CC_Strategy_and_Action_Plan_2022-2032_23_06_22_
ENGLISH-compressed.pdf
AU and NEPAD. (2003). New partnership for Africa's development: Action plan
for the environment initiative. https://www.nepad.org/publication/
action-plan-environment-initiative-0
AU and WHO. (2014). First meeting of African Ministers of Health jointly convened by the AUC and WHO. https://www.afro.who.int/sites/default/
files/2017-07/volume-1-ministerial-meeting-final-en.pdf
Hoogeveen, J. G., & Lopez-Acevedo, G. (2021, December 20). Distributional
impacts of COVID-19 in the Middle East and North Africa region. World
Bank Group. https://www.worldbank.org/en/region/mena/publication/
distributional-impacts-of-covid-19-in-the-middle-east-and-north-africa-region
OECD. (2020). COVID-19 in Africa: Regional socio-economic implications and
policy priorities. https://read.oecd-ilibrary.org/view/?ref=132_132745-
u5pt1rdb5x&title=COVID-19-in-Africa-Regional-socio-economic-
implications-and-policy-priorities
UNFCCC. (2014, September 25). Report of the conference of parties on its nine-
teenth session held in Warsaw from 11–13 November 2013. United Framework
Convention on Climate Change. https://unfccc.int/sites/default/files/
resource/docs/2013/cop19/eng/10a02r01.pdf
UNFCCC. (2022, November). Nationally determined contributions under the
Paris Agreement Synthesis report by the secretariat. United Nations Climate
Change. https://unfccc.int/documents/619180
WHO. (2021, October 30). Climate change and health. World Health
Organisation. https://www.who.int/news-room/fact-sheets/detail/climate-
change-and-health#:~:text=Between%202030%20and%202050%2C%20
climate,malaria%2C%20diarrhoea%20and%20heat%20stress
WHO & UNDP. (2018). Third Inter-Ministerial Conference on Health and
Environment in Africa: Conference Proceedings and Outcomes. https://wed-
ocs.unep.org/20.500.11822/33175
WHO & UNEP. (2008). The Libreville Declaration on Health and Environment
in Africa: 10 years on, 2008–2018. https://climhealthafrica.org/wp-content/
uploads/2020/05/2018-IMCHE3-THE-LIBREVILLE-DECLARATION-
ON-HEALTH-AND-ENVIRONMENT-IN-AFRICA-10-Years-
On-2008-2018.pdf

Health Data Sharing for Public Health Resilience: Benefits, Challenges, and Prospects in Africa

Henry Ngenyam Bang, Humphrey Ngala Ndi, and Emmanuel Etamo Kengo

INTRODUCTION

The phrase *"disease knows no borders"* reinvigorates the notion of vulnerability to the microbial world and encapsulates the risks posed by infectious diseases and pandemics in today's highly interconnected world.

H. N. Bang (✉)
Department of Disaster and Emergency Management,
Coventry University, Coventry, UK
e-mail: henry.bang@coventry.ac.uk

H. N. Ndi
High Commission for the Republic of Cameroon in London, London, UK

University of Yaounde I, Yaounde, Cameroon

E. E. Kengo
Department of History and African Civilizations, University of Buea,
Buea, Cameroon

© The Author(s), under exclusive license to Springer Nature   181
Switzerland AG 2023
H. N. Ndi et al. (eds.), *Health Diplomacy in Africa*, Studies in
Diplomacy and International Relations,
https://doi.org/10.1007/978-3-031-41249-3_9

Public health institutions, personnel, politicians, researchers, and academics have come to the painful reality that infectious diseases and viruses have the potential to easily spread across vast areas/regions within a short time. That could lead to international public health crises/emergencies like the ongoing COVID-19 pandemic that require intensive genomic monitoring efforts (Moodley et al., 2022). Indeed, infectious disease spread across vast geographical spaces is facilitated in regions where similar socio-economic and cultural drivers, epidemiological profiles, and regular travel of people and/or animals ease the transmission and sustenance of disease (Liverani et al., 2018). In such situations, there is a need for rapid sharing of data amongst scientists to facilitate surveillance and mitigate the effects (WHO, 2005).

Over the past few decades, infectious diseases that have posed cross-border risks like Zika in Latin America (Bogoch et al., 2016); avian influenza that occurred in Southeast Asia (Pfeiffer et al., 2011), and encephalitis in Japan. In Africa, there have been outbreaks of cholera in Sub-Saharan Africa (Bwire et al., 2016), onchocerciasis in West Africa (Gustavsen et al., 2016), and the prominent 2013–2016 Ebola epidemic in the West African region that affected Liberia, Sierra Leone, and Guinea due to the travel across the porous borders of these countries (Coltart et al., 2017; UNOCHA, 2015). Containing such disease spread is a priority for governments, public health officials/professionals, and scientists worldwide.

A common research practice has been for health researchers to protect their research findings for long durations until the data had been analysed and published (Nanda & Kowalczuk, 2014). Nevertheless, such practice is not in accordance with public health crises/emergencies when there is a grave threat to the lives and health of the world's populace (Juengst & Van Rie, 2020). To contain these infectious disease-induced global public health threats, there has been a paradigm shift in the way global health management agencies and frameworks tackle these health security risks. Sharing health data is now considered part of a comprehensive public health strategy to combat health crises, especially pandemics or easily transmitted diseases like the COVID-19 pandemic (GPA, 2021).

Under the auspices of the World Health Organization (WHO), International Health Regulations (IHR) were introduced to mitigate the spread of infectious diseases across international borders (Davies et al., 2015). The IHR stipulates that all countries and the international community have the responsibility to manage health crises resulting from infectious diseases. The guidance urges governments to enhance their public health potential and ability to detect, assess, monitor, and respond to impromptu disease outbreaks (WHO, 2005). Underpinned by rapid detection and response to incidents of infectious diseases, the IHRs enshrined global collaboration amongst agencies, institutions, and countries as critical for epidemic control (Davies & Youde, 2016). This laid a solid foundation for developing communication channels between health stakeholders and governments between and within countries worldwide.

Critical to the collaboration is the need to facilitate information/data sharing, sharing knowledge and expertise in disease control/management, ensuring routine surveillance of endemic diseases, expediting effective response during emergencies, and supporting ongoing work towards eliminating outbreaks (Gustavsen et al., 2016; Liverani et al., 2018). In accordance with the IHRs, several regional public health initiatives to enhance health data/information sharing have emerged around the world notably in Europe (Liverani & Coker, 2012), South America (Bruniera-Oliveira et al., 2017), Southeast Asia (Lover et al., 2016; Liverani et al., 2018), and Least and Medium Income Countries (LMIC) including in Africa (Ope et al., 2013). In consideration of the intrinsic impediments to electronic health data sharing, countries have been urged to consider the principles of proportionality, necessity, and effectiveness in processing people's data (GPA, 2021). Furthermore, some research funders have implemented a new criterion for researchers to share their raw data as a condition to receive funding (Bull et al., 2015; NIH Grants and Funding, 2020). How this is being received by African health researchers/academics is yet to be assessed.

Contemporary health research in Africa has been increasing with the potential to produce enormous datasets that can be invaluable to researchers working together to mitigate the high occurrence of disease in the continent (Rani & Buckley, 2012). While the sharing of health research information/data could enhance healthcare delivery in Africa, contemporary research shows that the practice is not yet common among healthcare agencies in the continent and is fraught with several challenges (Curley & Thomas, 2004; Thomas, 2006). We argue in this chapter that while data sharing is a key tool to combat communicable diseases in Africa and around the world, its limitations especially the challenges in data sharing need addressing urgently. Hence, there is a crucial requirement to explore the data-sharing activities of healthcare practitioners and researchers in Africa, which is the goal of this chapter.

The overarching aim of this chapter is to provide more clarity and understanding of the novel practice of international health data sharing with a focus on Africa. The three central objectives are to (1) understand the merits of health data sharing, (2) diagnose the challenges and impediments to health data sharing in Africa, and (3) suggest recommendations for enhancing health data sharing in African and LMICs.

The chapter contributes to enhancing health/epidemic risk reduction through international collaboration by increasing the literature on health data sharing. Policy, research, and academic scholarship on curbing infectious diseases through information will also benefit from the discourse in the chapter.

After the introduction, the next section is a succinct theoretical underpinning of health data sharing followed by a Section that discusses health data sharing policy from an international perspective. Next, is a Section that elaborates on the merits of sharing health data, followed by a discussion of the challenges and impediments to health data sharing. This leads to the last section, which is a combined conclusion, discussion, and recommendation on enhancing health data sharing in Africa.

DATA/INFORMATION SHARING: SUCCINCT CONCEPTUALIZATION

The central concept of interest in this chapter is the sharing of health-related data. Data sharing in the context of this chapter refers to making health data easily accessible to public authorities/agencies or other researchers/investigators locally, nationally, regionally, or internationally (Rowhani-Farid et al., 2017; IOM, 2015). Sources of the data could vary.

The data may be collected for research purposes by health research/medical agencies, organizations, institutions, or individual health researchers. Medical tests, or data collected by government agencies or other stakeholders like the health status of people during a pandemic fall into this category. This includes health data generated directly from the populace, patients, and clients, including demographic/survey data (Van-Panhuis et al., 2014). How the data is stored and disseminated matters.

Ideally, health data should be stored in regulated repositories that are safe and trusted and are able to be made available or shared with the various stakeholders without delay upon request (IOM, 2015). Data-sharing options range from open-access databases which do not have any restrictions to restricted databases (Van Noorden, 2021). In this digital era fuelled by advancements in information and communication technology, data sharing has been much easier, for instance, the use of data repositories has enabled academics/researchers to share data through digital object identifiers (DOI) (Rani & Buckley, 2012). Various research data/ dataset types can be shared including metadata, summary data, results on registries, publications, raw data, and cleaned datasets (IOM, 2015). Arguably, open science has the potential to foster research conduct that encourages standard processes/protocols for data sharing, dissemination, and reporting (Bierer et al., 2017). Ownership or control of databases has implications for how data is shared.

Data can be shared on both public and private online databases, public domain data science repositories, and regulated sharing initiatives like Global Initiative on Sharing Avian Influenza Data (GISAID). GISAID is a public-private partnership that has partnered with many countries and public health institutions/agencies around the world to share health data based on some core principles. The countries include the Federal Republic of Germany, China, South Africa, Singapore, Malaysia, the Republic of Congo, Brazil, Argentina, Ethiopia, Indonesia, Senegal, and Russia. GISAID is a novel initiative aimed to help researchers understand how viruses evolve and spread during epidemics and pandemics. It advocates for the rapid sharing of data from all influenza viruses, the coronavirus, and specific data associated with avian/animal viruses, including epidemiological/clinical data associated with human viruses' genetic sequence. Following weeks of the release of the first genomic data of the novel coronavirus on January 10, 2020, thousands of genomes were shared in GISAID, which was revolutionary, and it is notable that some African countries shared coronavirus data through it (Moodley et al., 2022). Nevertheless, how scientists feel about data sharing varies.

There has been contention on scientists' perception of accessing the databases. African health scientists have demanded adequate protection for collecting and sharing data while their European and North American counterparts have requested unrestricted access (Van Noorden, 2021; Maxmen, 2021). We contend, as discussed later in this chapter, that the approach to database access from African health scientists is not unrelated to the challenges they have been facing while collaborating with their peers in Western countries.

HEALTH DATA SHARING POLICY/GUIDELINES

The sharing and reuse of data can be of enormous benefit to public health and scientific research generally. In public health, data sharing enables a better understanding of health issues and evidence-informed decisions taking. As the leading actor in global health management, the WHO launched a new policy and guidelines that necessitates sharing of cross-border research data between countries in emergency and non-emergency situations (WHO, 2007). Known as the IHRs, countries in different regions of the world are encouraged to forge a closer partnership to mitigate vulnerabilities from infectious diseases. In fact, Article 57 of the IHR states that States should support *"bilateral or multilateral agreements or arrangements across countries"* to foster joint action, including the direct and rapid exchange of public health information between neighbouring territories of different States" (WHO, 2005).

The WHO guidelines in public health surveillance, which addresses ethical issues during public health crises recommend that during a public health emergency, it is important that stakeholders involved in surveillance should share data in a timely manner (WHO, 2017). The policy encapsulates the reuse of health data on research grounds with an emphasis that the data will be used in an efficient, ethical, and equitable manner (WHO, 2022). The WHO believes this policy will enhance its goal of providing one billion more people with better health and well-being. Other international organizations and countries are incorporating data sharing into their policies.

In November 2021, UNESCO released a document containing a draft recommendation on global data sharing of science, technology, and innovation with the objective to *"...provide an international framework for Open Science policy and practice..."* (UNESCO, 2021). Data sharing has also been considered at the government level, for instance, the United States requires that research funded by the Federal Government must be shared (National Academy of Sciences, Engineering, and Medicine, 2015). Furthermore, sharing research data is increasingly being considered a criterion for research funding, including the funding of medical research.

For example, sharing data has been inculcated into the WHO's research funding requirement (WHO, 2022) and many funders of public health research now require unrestricted data sharing (Kadakia et al., 2021). Funding Bodies like the Wellcome Trust, The Bill and Melinda Gates Foundation, and The National Institute of Health (NIH) now require researchers to share their data as a precondition for funding (Bull et al., 2015; NIH Grants and Funding, 2020). Indeed, the Research Council UK (RCUK) supports funded research and its guidance on best practices in the management of research data states that *"Publicly funded research data are a public good, produced in the public interest...and should be openly available to the maximum extent possible"* (RCUK, 2015, p1–2). Open data is data that is easily accessible, intelligible, discoverable, assessable, useable and if possible, interoperable to certain standards while respecting safety, security and privacy concerns, and commercial interests (ibid). Some research, academic and professional journals now require that data be shared as a condition for papers to be published (National Academy of Sciences, Engineering, and Medicine, 2015).

In developing data sharing policy, the competent authorities should ensure it has public trust by protecting privacy. Building public confidence/trust in travel health data requires that some conditions be fulfilled: the required data is not too much, the data is kept safely, the purpose for processing the data is known, how the data shall be used is understood, and the data will not be kept longer than necessary (WHO, 2005, 2007). Furthermore, a plan for sharing and managing data is essential for effective data sharing. The WHO has provided operational guidance that has ethical, technical, and legal considerations on how researchers can develop and implement a plan for data management and sharing. The guidance on data sharing for secondary analysis provides advice that does not compromise the privacy of patients (WHO, 2022).

We have compiled some good principles for processing health data for the purposes of international travel that align with global data protection. These are outlined below:

- Health data must only be processed when required or if necessary.
- All health data sharing systems and/or processes including data sharing arrangements for international travel should embed the principles of *"Privacy by design and default"*.
- Prior to processing the health data, it is vital to initially carry out a risk assessment of the impact on the populace and/or communities that supplied the data.
- All the responsible agencies/organizations tasked with health data collection/processing should function under the auspices of an appropriate government authority or recognized agencies/institutions.

- In view of protecting public health, the responsible agencies should collect the minimum health information from people or from other legal sources.
- People have the right to know how their data shall be used, those to use it and the specific purposes for demanding the data. This information should be concisely and clearly communicated to the populace in recognition of linguistic, cultural, and geographical diversity.
- The data collection purpose should be made public and clearly explained within the public health measures at the time.
- While it is justifiable to process health data for international travel based on protecting public health, it is vital that risks to personal privacy should be considered at the onset.
- The responsible agencies should consider the time or duration for retaining an individual's health data and come up with a programme for deleting data once it is no longer needed.
- Governments should consider the data protection rights of vulnerable people. These include individuals who lack access to electronic devices or are unable to use them and people with peculiar underlying health risks/conditions.
- The health authorities should be conscious of the risks involved in sharing health records for the purpose of international travel.
- Data sharing via digital systems comes with cybersecurity risks. Hence it is necessary to investigate or assess the tools such as apps that are popularly used for sharing data.
- A review of health data sharing should be done periodically to ensure subsequent data processing is appropriate in view of the evolving health crises (GPA, 2021; Ferber et al., 2016; WHO, 2005, 2007, 2022; Ottenbacher et al., 2019; UNESCO, 2021).

Data sharing for travel was predominant during the coronavirus pandemic. Indeed, the pandemic demonstrated the relevance of privacy by design in public health data sharing on a mass scale for travel. Elements of health information such as COVID-19 test results, vaccination status, and health passports were either used or proposed by governments. The scale and speed of the data sharing were facilitated by digital technology (GPA, 2021).

Merits of Sharing Health Data

Emphasis on data sharing and the merits of sharing health data nationally, regionally, and internationally cannot be overemphasized. The literature has a satisfactory assessment of the benefits of efficient and widespread sharing of health data including, but not limited to the following:

- Promote expanded scientific inquiry with the potential to improve public health.
- Facilitates resolving global health crises and/or emergencies.
- Enhances scientific/research skills/innovation and boosts the application of knowledge to health policies, programmes, and products.
- Enables more people in the world to have access to better well-being and health.
- Has the ability to create innovations in data management including its collection, analysis, and validation.
- Data sharing aids to inform policy decisions/interventions on health issues.
- Enable researchers, empower citizens and convey academic, economic, and social benefits.
- Encourages transparent, open, and robust research.
- Increase more reuse of data, facilitates data combination from multiple datasets, and motivate wider data analysis.
- Increases avenues for scientific collaboration, alliances, and cooperation.
- Enables the data to be reproducible, replicable, comprehensible, and verifiable with the view to encourage open science.
- Promotes honesty, public trust, completeness, accountability, and sincerity among health practitioners in scientific research.
- Increase avenues for public transparency and engagement.
- Merging datasets has the potential to generate substantial statistical proficiency and grant potential opportunities for comparative research.
- Strengthen performance measures and assessment capacity.
- Improve and expedite the discovery of health risks with implications for improving research into options and tracking of instantaneous responses.

- Strengthen research standards by reducing duplication of research.
- When data sharing is combined across time and countries/regions it could provide answers to new/emerging questions and be cost-effective including saving time and effort (RCUK, 2015; Rowhani-Farid et al., 2017; Loveth et al., 2022; Huston et al., 2019; Ferber et al., 2016; Ottenbacher et al., 2019; Pisani et al., 2010).

The COVID-19 pandemic can be used to illustrate the advantages of health data sharing. The early detection and speedy sharing of information regarding suspicious variants as the pandemic raged, enabled vaccine companies to use genomic data to modify their vaccines. This enabled the omicron-adapted coronavirus vaccine to be distributed across North America and the European Union in time for the anticipated rise in infections (Moodley et al., 2022). In addition, sharing data openly with researchers, scientists, health research agencies, or governments during the pandemic helped in the development of diagnostic kits, and vaccines, and expedited any innovative mitigation, preparedness, or response strategies needed (Juengst & Van Rie, 2020).

Other than the points mentioned above, sharing of health information in Africa adds to public health value (Ope et al., 2013) and in addition, helps in strengthening cooperation among African countries, especially in the collective development of research skills, technical expertise, and knowledge exchange (UNDP, 2007).

Some researchers have recommended that best practices in sharing data require the involvement of a brokering agency to perform some key tasks. These include creating viable channels of communication between countries, rectifying disparities in the data-sharing process between partners in different countries and maximizing health datasets/information (Liverani et al., 2018). We would argue that this could be useful in circumstances where some or all the agencies involved are not experienced or knowledgeable in data-sharing practices or modalities. Nevertheless, the interest of the brokering agency must be clear. If they have financial interests in the deal, that could compromise the integrity of the role in the data-sharing process which could raise moral and/or ethical issues and could instead pose an impediment to the data sharing.

The State of Health Data Sharing in Africa

Whereas the African Union has always cherished health data sharing in the interest of cross-border disease surveillance, no such sharing takes place on a routine basis. Generally, some form of cross-border health cooperation only occurs when a disease of epidemic or pandemic potential breaks out in a neighbouring country. Even so, it is never an easy, fast, and straightforward thing. One of the obstacles is the absence of internationally endorsed protocols to ensure that crucial health information is shared immediately and in intelligible forms wherever and whenever an outbreak occurs (Yozwiak et al., 2015). The most palpable case is that of the West African Ebola Virus Disease (EVD) epidemic between 2013 and 2015. Data-sharing barriers were innumerable as the ministries of health of the most affected countries (Guinea, Liberia, and Sierra Leone) tended to share the relevant data through the WHO rather than directly among themselves (Georgetown University Medical Center, 2018). The failure to share health data in a timely manner has been cited as one of the main obstacles to effective EVD response.

An efficient and quick flow of information across borders is, therefore, crucial for averting such incidents of cross-border spread. The African Union (AU) Data Policy Framework, which should provide the contexts and procedures for data sharing, was created in February 2022, less than a year ago. This framework follows many previous attempts at data governance on the continent starting with the Addis Ababa Plan of Action for Statistical Development in Africa of 1990.

Its goal is to strengthen information systems that support public health strategies in Africa. One of the strategies is to design and implement a continental data-sharing platform for Member States by linking public health institutes in each country through a wide area network managed by the Africa Centre of Disease Control (CDC). This will enhance the secure electronic transmission of relevant data and reports, enable data queries, and provide dashboard reporting to monitor priority objectives and outbreak responses. The network may support functional regional networks within the Wide Area Network (WAN). The framework also aims to organize, convene, and support working groups to develop and promote network domains as well as the adoption of informatics guidelines and standards to enable interconnectivity and electronic transmission of data and information among Africa CDC institutes; support training through the Regional Collaborating Centres (RCC) on informatics such as geographic information systems, network domains, analytical and management software, and hardware, including functional needs assessments and procurement; and establish data observatories at Africa CDC, RCCs through training and collaboration.

The Africa CDC initiative to create five regional integrated surveillance and laboratory networks (RISLNET) is intended to improve surveillance and control of high-priority endemic or neglected diseases on the continent. The World Bank approved the project in 2020 with the aim to support the Africa CDC to bolster continental and regional infectious disease detection and response systems. A subcomponent of the network will be the establishment of a small number of fit-for-purpose laboratories, and transnational surveillance networks which include data sharing, emergency-response mechanisms, and other health assets designed to manage disease risks on a regional or continental scale.

When established, RISLNET will leverage existing regional public health assets including the surveillance and laboratory networks operated by public agencies, private organizations, foundations, and universities to create an integrated electronic network of regional surveillance platforms.

The proposed project will lead to the development of an incorporated information technology platform and infrastructure for connecting RCCs and NPHIs; transportation and processing of samples for testing at Africa CDC-affiliated laboratories in Ethiopia and Zambia; the procurement of reagents and specialized materials for sample testing; and technical assistance for the operationalization of RISLNET bureaus in Eastern and Southern Africa. The subcomponent will also support the Africa CDC in developing innovative information-sharing systems and establishing itself as a trusted source of health information through the Extension for Community Health Outcomes (ECHO) platform, which uses videoconferencing and structured case presentations to develop virtual communities of practice. The five RISLNET in view shall be located in Northern Africa, Western Africa, Central Africa, Eastern Africa, and Southern Africa.

Challenges in Data Sharing in Africa

Contemporary research shows that health data circulation has increased across international borders. This was also evident during the coronavirus pandemic albeit with challenges in resource-poor countries. There are several reasons for the reluctance or low frequency of sharing health research data, or why the data is withheld in Africa. These include, but are not limited to the following:

- The similarities and differences between the national health sectors of countries.
- Diversity of regional health activities.
- Limited capacity within countries and capacity gaps between less- and more-resourced States.
- Weak legislative and institutional frameworks to sustain regional cooperation amongst partners.
- Complex state politics.
- Lack of or insufficient motivation for sharing data.
- There are unequal research resource and infrastructure inequalities between Northern and Southern countries.
- The historical context of Western exploitation of Africa and the tendency for data to be generated in Africa and the analysis to be done in developed countries creates issues of power equality between researchers.
- Unfunded research costs are high for individual researchers.
- Issues with data confidentiality and quality, including data-sharing skills.
- Data ownership and community relevance.
- Lack of consensus among scientists on how data should be shared. For instance, the anonymity and protection of data contributors have been criticized and some critics prefer public-domain repositories.
- Digital technology that provides opportunities for data sharing is still developing in Africa and is yet to be fully understood by users.
- Researchers in Africa do not receive enough credit for work done through collaborative research with their peers in Western countries.
- Disproportionate distribution of gains derived from data sharing.
- There are implications for public perceptions of data sharing that would lead to measures that will adversely affect the populace.
- Data analysis skills/expertise are unevenly distributed with more capacity/resources in Western/Northern countries than in Southern countries (National Academy of Sciences, Engineering and Medicine, 2015; De Vries et al., 2011; Thomas, 2006; Hameiri, 2014; Liverani et al., 2018; Moodley, 2020).

Our analysis shows that legal, political, ethical, financial, technical, and socio-cultural factors are responsible for the reluctance or impediments to data sharing in Africa. Of peculiar attention is the fact that different rules guide the movement of health data within and outside countries, there are a variety of standards/practices in different countries, language barriers impact data sharing/communication, issues exist with sustaining financial arrangements, and disparity in human resource abilities and capacities (Liverani et al., 2018). In addition, enormous resources, effort, skill, and competence are required for collecting, processing, storing, disseminating, sharing, and managing data, which is limited in resource-limited African countries (Bull et al., 2015; Van-Panhuis et al., 2014; Mello et al., 2013). Ethical reasons include worries regarding the ability of some researchers to ensure the confidentiality/anonymity of data (Mello et al., 2013), especially in circumstances where the probability of some participants being recognized is increased due to the merging of datasets (Bull et al., 2015). How the public perceives data sharing influences attitudes toward data sharing. For instance, Keymanthri et al. (2022) found that people's negative feelings about data sharing have made them refuse consent to subsequent sharing of data.

We have used specific incidents, case studies, or examples to further diagnose the challenges faced by African countries in data collaboration and sharing. While data sharing is not yet common practice among health researchers or their agencies in Africa (Bezuidenhout & Chakauya, 2018), several contextual issues in data sharing practice deter African health researchers from sharing data (Anane-Sarpong et al., 2018) as highlighted above. A few case studies are discussed in the following paragraphs.

During the COVID-19 pandemic, efforts at data sharing led to many southern African countries being unjustly ostracized (Seydi, 2021). This was experienced when South Africa alerted the world to the new omicron virus strand and shared data on genomic sequencing of the omicron variant. The country was immediately banned from international travel to Northern countries although it did not derive any benefit from alerting the international community. Instead, the travel restrictions had moral and economic consequences for the region and seriously affected progress in South Africa's research since researchers could not receive laboratory equipment due to the ban (Moodley et al., 2022). Furthermore, the scientists were rebuked by local communities for sharing the omicron virus genomic data that was used to implement restrictive travel measures that affected them (Mallapaty, 2021). Nevertheless, the travel restrictions had a limited impact on the spread of the disease to other continents (Keymanthri et al., 2022).

A point worth mentioning is that researchers from Northern and Southern countries benefit disproportionately from joined research. Arguably, there are no adequate international ethical principles on the legality of data sharing or how African countries and their local researchers and communities that supply health data would equally benefit from joined research where data is shared between the North and the South. For example, during the Ebola outbreak, an estimated 50,000 samples were illegally taken out of Africa without consent or export permits (Schroeder et al., 2019). This requires urgent action to stop this unethical practice.

Another issue that is worth highlighting is the fact that the contribution of African research to global scientific innovation or discovery is often undermined. This is evidenced in the discovery of the Ebola virus where sole credit was given to one scientist, Dr Peter Piot (a Belgian microbiologist) although his African colleague, Dr Jean-Jacques Muyembe Tamfum (a Congolese microbiologist) sent him the blood samples used to isolate the virus (Branswel, 2016).

The lack of adequate representation at the governance level of global databases is another factor. For instance, many independent organizations or agencies govern the GISAID database, which has been very popular and instrumental over the past decade in storing and sharing health data (Moodley et al., 2022). Nevertheless, Longo and Drazen (2016) assert that the database has no representatives from Africa although it contains enormous data that has been contributed by African researchers. We think this is an oversight and this mistake should be rectified to ensure the governance structure has global representation.

A history of exploitation in research practices in sharing data has also been identified as a limitation to data sharing in Africa. It is an open secret that vaccine access for LMICs has always been limited albeit some countries have contended patents on medication and vaccines developed from data that had been acquired freely from shared collaboration. Another example of resistance borne out of exploitation happened in 2007 when Indonesia refused requests to share samples of the H5N1 virus with the WHO after officials were informed that an Australian pharmaceutical company had plans to use the samples to develop a vaccine. The refusal was informed by Indonesia's previous poor experience with the unethical use of its data after making it available to WHO's Global Influenza Surveillance Network (Moodley et al., 2022). This shows a lack of trust in sharing research data, which could have dire consequences for subsequent cooperation, as revealed by this incident.

Despite the challenges in data sharing in Africa, it is comforting to note that African countries and their health/academic institution have realized the need to jointly address the issue through various methods. For instance, a workshop on the benefits of and barriers to sharing research data to improve public health in Africa was held from March 29 to 30, 2015, in South Africa (National Academy of Sciences, Engineering, and Medicine, 2015). The African Union established the data policy framework which should provide the contexts and procedures for data sharing on the continent in February 2022.

Conclusion, Discussion, and Recommendation

This chapter has discussed the concept of health data sharing with keen attention to Africa. The discourse has addressed key underpinning issues in health data sharing such as the concept of data sharing, data-sharing policies/guidelines, and the merits and challenges plaguing health data sharing in Africa. Prominent in the discourse is the benefits of and barriers to sharing health data with the overarching aim to enhance the resilience of global public health from infectious diseases.

The advantages of health data sharing and making research data openly and freely available, accessible, and reusable have been underscored, not least as a practice that demonstrates research integrity. Yet, the process of achieving this still rests on individual institutional capacities (Bezuidenhout & Chakauya, 2018). An international and/or joined framework between Northern and Southern countries to improve data sharing would be relevant to facilitate the process. From the analysis in this chapter, we have concluded that sharing health data for research purposes that are beneficial to public health, especially to mitigate international health crises is undoubtedly necessary, not least from a scientific perspective.

This chapter highlights the complex socio-technical nature of data and information sharing in Africa, where health decision-making is becoming more complex, with the implication that health data sharing has not been firmly established in resource-poor economies. Despite global encouragement for data sharing, analysis in this chapter has revealed significant barriers to data collection and sharing in Africa. These are rooted in unique cultural, financial, political, legal, ethical, technical, moral, social, and economic situations which arguably are beyond the capacity of the scientific community to easily resolve (Anane-Sarpong et al., 2020). We would argue that the challenges and negative consequences associated with sharing data demotivate and discourage transparency in African researchers. It is also responsible for the lukewarm attitude or lack of enthusiasm among southern health researchers for sharing research information beyond their established networks or collaborations (National Academy of Sciences, Engineering, and Medicine, 2015)

From the identified challenges, we recommend that the sharing of health data should be done responsibly with moral considerations and social justice as core principles to be considered. This would avoid disproportionate benefits from the various research stakeholders and avoid inequality.

Furthermore, lessons should be learned from the negative social and economic consequences of the international travel ban on South Africa following the omicron variant genome sequencing announcement. Local reactions to this incident can be likened to the fact that the South African researchers *"shot themselves in the foot"* by revealing the new virus strain, which was used to sanction their country. Although they acted in good faith for the good of international public health, they may be reluctant to report similar emerging diseases in the future, with implications for subsequent cooperation in health data sharing. This would be ironic in the sense that the main risk to future data sharing/disclosure could result from sharing data.

During the discussion, we highlighted gaps in data sharing with suggested means of containing them. Further recommendations are mentioned below:

- Research networks and collaborations between rich and poor countries should include research teams who collect/generate and share data.
- African health research institutions should empower African researchers to develop a sustainable research surveillance and data-sharing culture.
- Agencies, organizations, or research institutions tasked with health data collection, processing and sharing must operate under the auspices of a recognized government authority and should be regulated.
- Governance of global research databases like GISAID should have representatives from Africa to reflect global inclusiveness in its management.
- More stringent enforceable and binding policies should be developed that support the right of all stakeholders to equally benefit from sharing health data.

- Community perception of data sharing should not be ignored. Local communities and the populace should be sensitized to understand the public health benefits of sharing data.
- Change in the global research data-sharing frameworks is necessary to promote an enabling research culture that will remove inequality and provide greater participation from African researchers.
- To facilitate data sharing, African countries, with assistance from their western partners, enhance their information and communication (ICT) technology infrastructure in consideration of the invaluable role that digital technology plays in sharing health data worldwide.
- Adequate governance mechanisms for open data sharing are necessary and should be harmonized to avoid discrimination or disproportionality in research teams from poor and rich countries.
- Mechanisms should be put in place to regularly communicate data-sharing practices to the public.
- Principles of social responsibility, social justice, and equality should be embedded in data-sharing principles to ensure that the rights, values, equality, and interest of both the data collection teams and the local populace are respected.
- The concept of data authorship, which has emerged to ensure that researchers who generate data are acknowledged in publications (Bierer et al., 2017) should be implemented.
- Decisions that are derived from data collected from a specific population, which could adversely affect that population should be seriously considered and the least severe measures should be taken.
- Public health decisions should incorporate the principles of social justice, solidarity, efficiency, and proportionality.
- In implementing international public health measures, African countries should carefully gauge the socio-economic impact on their populace.

Hopefully, the issues, challenges, and suggested recommendations discussed in this chapter will contribute to enhancing health data sharing in the future. The discourse has addressed a contemporary and topical public health issue with great potential to inform literature in the field including national/international policy development which could improve North-South cooperation in health data sharing.

REFERENCES

Anane-Sarpong, E., Wangmo, T., & Tanner, M. (2020). Ethical principles for promoting health research data sharing with sub-Saharan Africa. *Developing World Bioethics, 20*(2), 86–95. https://doi.org/10.1111/dewb.12233

Anane-Sarpong, E., Wangmo, T., Ward, C., Sankoh, T., Tanner, M., & Elger, B. (2018). You cannot collect data using your own resources and put it on open access: Perspectives from Africa about public health data-sharing. *Developing World Bioethics, 18*(4), 394–405. https://doi.org/10.1111/dewb.12159

Bezuidenhout, L., & Chakauya, E. (2018). Hidden concerns of sharing research data by low/middle-income country scientists. *Global Bioethics, 29*(1), 39–54. https://doi.org/10.1080/11287462.2018.1441780

Bierer, E., Crosas, M., & Pierce, H. (2017). Data authorship as an incentive for data sharing. *New England Journal of Medicine, 377*(4), 402. https://doi.org/10.1056/NEJMc1707245

Bogoch, I., Brady, O., Kraemer, G., German, M., Creatore, M., Kulkarni, M., Brownstein, J., Mekaru, S., Hay, S., Groot, E., Watts, E., & Khan, W. (2016). Anticipating the international spread of Zika virus from Brazil. *The Lancet, 387*(10016), 335–336. https://doi.org/10.1016/S0140-6736(16)00080-5

Branswel, H. (2016, July 14). History credits this man with discovering Ebola on his own. History is wrong. *Statnews*. https://www.statnews.com/2016/07/14/history-ebola-peter-piot/

Bruniera-Oliveira, R., Horta, P., Varan, A., Montiel, S., Carmo, H., Waterman, H., & Verani, J. (2017). Epidemiological surveillance of land borders in North and South America: A case study. *Revista Instituto Medican Tropical Sao Paulo, 59.* https://doi.org/10.1590/S1678-9946201759068

Bull, S., Roberts, N., & Parker, M. (2015). Views of ethical best practices in sharing individual-level data from medical and public health research: A systematic scoping review. *Journal of Empirical Research on Human Research Ethics, 10*(3), 225–238. https://doi.org/10.1177/1556264615594767

Bwire, G., Mwesawina, M., Baluku, Y., Kanyanda, S., & Orach, G. (2016). Cross-border cholera outbreaks in sub-Saharan Africa, the mystery behind the silent illness: What needs to be done? *PLoS One, 11*(6), e0156674. https://doi.org/10.1371/journal.pone.0156674

Coltart, C., Lindsey, B., Ghinai, I., Johnson, A., & Heymann, D. (2017). The Ebola outbreak, 2013–2016: Old lessons for new epidemics. *Philosophical Transactions of the Royal Society, 372*(1721), 20160297. https://doi.org/10.1098/rstb.2016.0297

Curley, M., & Thomas, N. (2004). Human security and public health in Southeast Asia: The SARS outbreak. *Australian Journal of International Affairs, 58*(1), 17–32. https://doi.org/10.1080/1035771032000184737

Davies, E., Kamradt-Scott, A., & Rushton, S. (2015). *Disease diplomacy: International norms and global health security.* Johns Hopkins University Press.

Davies, E., & Youde, J. (2016). *The politics of surveillance and response to disease outbreaks: The new frontier for states and non-state actors.* Routledge.

De Vries, J., Bull, S. J., Doumbo, O., Ibrahim, M., Mercereau-Puijalon, O., Kwiatkowski, D., & Parker, M. (2011). Ethical issues in human genomics research in developing countries. *BMC Medical Ethics, 12*(5). https://doi.org/10.1186/1472-6939-12-5

Ferber, R., Osis, S., Hicks, J., & Delp, L. (2016). Gait biomechanics in the era of data science. *Journal of Biomechanics, 49*(16), 3759–3761. https://doi.org/10.1016/j.jbiomech.2016.10.033

Georgetown University Medical Center. (2018). *Data sharing during the West Africa Ebola public health emergency: Case study report.* Georgetown University.

GPA. (2021). GPA executive committee joint statement on the use of health data for domestic or international travel purposes. https://globalprivacyassembly.org/gpa-executive-committee-joint-statement-on-the-use-of-health-data-for-domestic-or-international-travel-purposes/

Gustavsen, K., Sodahlon, Y., & Bush, S. (2016). Cross-border collaboration for neglected tropical disease efforts-lessons learned from onchocerciasis control and elimination in the Mano River Union (West Africa). *Global Health, 12*(1), 44. https://doi.org/10.1186/s12992-016-0185-5

Hameiri, S. (2014). Avian influenza, 'viral sovereignty', and the politics of health security in Indonesia. *The Pacific Review, 27*(3), 333–356. https://doi.org/10.1080/09512748.2014.909523

Huston, P., Edge, V., & Bernier, E. (2019). Reaping the benefits of open data in public health. *Canadian Communicable Disease Report, 45*(11), 252–256. https://doi.org/10.14745/ccdr.v45i10a0

IOM. (2015). *Sharing clinical trial data: Maximizing benefits, minimizing risk.* The National Academics Press.

Juengst, E., & Van Rie, A. (2020). Transparency, trust, and community welfare: Towards a precision public health ethics framework for the genomics era. *Genome Medicine, 12*, 98. https://doi.org/10.1186/s13073-020-00800-y

Kadakia, K., Beckman, A., Ross, J., & Krumholz, M. (2021). Leveraging open science to accelerate research. *New England Journal of Medicine, 384*(17). https://doi.org/10.1056/NEJMp2034518

Keymanthri, M., Nezerith, C., Aneeka, D., Gonasagrie, N., Adetayo, E., & Lessells, R. (2022). Ethics and governance challenges related to genomic data sharing in southern Africa: The case of SARS-CoV-2. *The Lancet, 10*(12). https://doi.org/10.1016/S2214-109X(22)00417-X

Liverani, M., & Coker, R. (2012). Protecting Europe from diseases: From the international sanitary conferences to the ECDC. *Journal of Health Politics Policy Law, 37*(6), 915–934. https://doi.org/10.1215/03616878-1813772

Liverani, M., Teng, S., Le, M., & Coker, R. (2018). Sharing public health data and information across borders: Lessons from Southeast Asia. *Global Health, 14*, 94. https://doi.org/10.1186/s12992-018-0415-0

Longo, D., & Drazen, M. (2016). Data sharing. *New England Journal of Medicine, 374*, 276–277. https://doi.org/10.1056/NEJMe1516564

Lover, A., Gosling, R., Feachem, R., & Tulloch, J. (2016). Eliminate now: Seven critical actions required to accelerate elimination of plasmodium falciparum malaria in the greater Mekong subregion. *Malaria Journal, 15*(1), 518. https://doi.org/10.1186/s12936-016-1564-3

Loveth, O., Benita, O., Agnes, S., & Aletha, W. (2022). Data sharing practices of health researchers in Africa: A scoping review protocol. *JBI Evidence Synthesis, 20*(2), 681–688. https://doi.org/10.11124/JBIES-20-00502

Mallapaty, S. (2021). Omicron-variant border bans ignore the evidence, say scientists. *Nature, 600*, 199. https://www.icpcovid.com/sites/default/files/2021-12/Eppercent201974percent20Omicronvariantpercent20borderpercent20banspercent20ignorepercent20thepercent20evidencepercent2Cpercent20saypercent20scientists.pdf

Maxmen, A. (2021). Why some researchers oppose unrestricted sharing of coronavirus genome data. *Nature, 593*, 176–177. https://doi.org/10.1038/d41586-021-01194-6

Mello, M., Francer, J., Wilenzick, M., Teden, P., Bierer, B., & Barnes, M. (2013). Preparing for responsible sharing of clinical trial data. *New England Journal of Medicine, 369*(17), 1651–1658. https://doi.org/10.1056/NEJMhle1309073

Moodley, K. (2020). Research imperialism resurfaces in South Africa in the midst of the COVID-19 pandemic—This time, via a digital portal. *South African Medical Journal, 110*(11), 1068–1069. https://doi.org/10.7196/samj.2020.v110i11.15285

Moodley, N., Domingo, A., Nair, G., Obasa, A., Lessells, R., & Oliveira, T. (2022). Ethics and governance challenges related to genomic data sharing in southern Africa: The case of SARS-CoV-2. *The Lancet, 10*(12), 1855–1859. https://doi.org/10.1016/S2214-109X(22)00417-X

Nanda, S., & Kowalczuk, M. (2014). Unpublished genomic data–how to share? *BMC Genomics, 15*, 5. https://doi.org/10.1186/1471-2164-15-5

National Academy of Sciences, Engineering and Medicine. (2015). *Sharing research data to improve public health in Africa. A workshop summary.* The National Academies Press. https://www.nia.nih.gov/sites/default/files/2017-06/sharing-research-data-to-improve-public-health-in-africa_0.pdf

NIH Grants and Funding. (2020). NIH data sharing policy and implementation guidance. https://grants.nih.gov/grants/policy/data_sharing/data_sharing_guidance.htm

Ope, M., Sonoiya, S., Kariuki, J., Mboera, L., Gandham, R., Schneidman, M., & Kimura, M. (2013). Regional initiatives in support of surveillance in East

Africa: The East Africa integrated disease surveillance network (EAIDSNet) experience. *Emergency Health Threats Journal*, 6(1). https://doi.org/10.3402/ehtj.v6i0.19948

Ottenbacher, K., Graham, J., & Fisher, S. (2019). Data science in physical medicine and rehabilitation: Opportunities and challenges. *Physical Medicine and Rehabilitation Clinics*, 30(2), 459–471. https://doi.org/10.1016/j.pmr.2018.12.003

Pfeiffer, D., Otte, J., Roland-Holst, D., Inui, K., Nguyen, T., & Zilberman, D. (2011). Implications of global and regional patterns of highly pathogenic avian influenza virus H5N1 clades for risk management. *The Veterinary Journal*, 190(3), 309–316. https://doi.org/10.1016/j.tvjl.2010.12.022

Pisani, E., Whitworth, J., Zaba, B., & Abou-Zahr, C. (2010). Time for fair trade in research data. *Lancet*, 375(9716), 703–705. https://doi.org/10.1016/S0140-6736(09)61486-0

Rani, M., & Buckley, S. (2012). Systematic archiving and access to health research data: Rationale, current status and way forward. *Bulletin of the World Health Organisation*, 90, 932–939. https://doi.org/10.2471/blt.12.105908

RCUK. (2015). Guidance on best practice in the management of research data. https://www.ukri.org/wp-content/uploads/2020/10/UKRI-020920-GuidanceBestPracticeManagementResearchData.pdf

Rowhani-Farid, A., Allen, M., & Barnett, G. (2017). What incentives increase data sharing in health and medical research? A systematic review. *Research Integrity and Peer Review*, 2(1), 4. https://doi.org/10.1186/s41073-017-0028-9

Schroeder, D., Chatfield, K., Singh, M., Chennells, R., & Herissone-Kelly, P. (2019). Exploitation risks in collaborative international research. In D. Schroeder, K. Chatfield, M. Singh, R. Chennells, & P. Herissone-Kelly (Eds.), *Equitable research partnerships* (pp. 37–50). Springer. https://doi.org/10.1007/978-3-030-15745-6_5

Seydi, O. (2021). Southern Africa: Last in line for vaccines, first in line for travel bans. https://fortune.com/2021/12/09/south-africa-vaccines-travel-ban-omicron-pandemic-variant-covid-oumar-seydi/

Thomas, N. (2006). The regionalization of avian influenza in East Asia: Responding to the next pandemic(?). *Asian Survey*, 46(6), 917–936. https://doi.org/10.1525/as.2006.46.6.917

UNDP. (2007). Evaluation of UNDP contribution to south-south cooperation. New York: United Nations Development Programme. http://web.undp.org/evaluation/documents/thematic/ssc/SSC_Evaluation.pdf

UNESCO. (2021). First draft of the UNESCO recommendation on Open Science. https://en.unesco.org/sites/default/files/comments_osr_partner_osi_document.pdf

UNOCHA. (2015). Strengthening border surveillance between Ebola affected countries. Ebola Bulletin. https://www.humanitarianresponse.info/sites/www.humanitarianresponse.info/files/documents/files/ebola_hb_18_july_final.pdf

Van Noorden, R. (2021). Scientists call for fully open sharing of coronavirus genome data. Nature, 590(7845), 195–196. https://doi.org/10.1038/d41586-021-00305-7

Van-Panhuis, W., Proma, P., Emerson, C., Grefenstette, J., Wilder, R., Herbst, A., Heymann, D., & Burke, D. (2014). A systematic review of barriers to data sharing in public health. BMC Public Health, 14(1), 1144. https://doi.org/10.1186/1471-2458-14-1144

WHO. (2005). International health regulations 2005. https://www.who.int/health-topics/international-health-regulations#tab=tab_1

WHO. (2007, February 26–28). Cross-border collaboration on emerging infectious diseases. Report of the bi-regional meeting Bangkok. WHO Regional Office for Southeast Asia. https://apps.who.int/iris/bitstream/handle/10665/204925/B0632.pdf?sequence=1

WHO. (2017). The WHO guidelines on ethical issues in public health surveillance. World Health Organization, Geneva. https://www.who.int/publications/i/item/who-guidelines-on-ethical-issues-in-public-health-surveillance

WHO. (2022). New WHO policy requires sharing of all research data. https://www.who.int/news/item/16-09-2022-new-who-policy-requires-sharing-of-all-research-data

Yozwiak, N. L., Schaffner, S. F., & Sabeti, P. C. (2015). Data sharing: Make outbreak research open access. Nature, 518(7540), 477–479. https://doi.org/10.1038/518477a

CHAPTER 10

With or Without Diplomacy: The Urgent Need to Decolonize Healthcare in Africa

Godfrey B. Tangwa

INTRODUCTION

It is important for me to start this chapter by recommending a radical mental decolonization and reform of concepts and expressions likely to cover up or to obscure what needs critical examination and redressing, in the healthcare situation in Africa.

We urgently need decolonizing our minds (Wa Thiong'o, 1992; Wiredu, 1997) and the concepts and terms that we are habituated to use unthinkingly or uncritically. We must abandon terms and concepts imposed without justification from our own point of view and perspective by colonialism, neo-colonialism, and the colonial legacy. These terms and concepts have had a long evolution and basically consider and look on Africa and Africans as a colonial asset and an economic resource to be guiltlessly wantonly exploited. Many Africans unconsciously use and apply these concepts and terms without knowing their historical evolution necessitated by

G. B. Tangwa (✉)
University of Yaounde 1, Yaounde, Cameroon

Cameroon Bioethics Initiative (CAMBIN), Yaounde, Cameroon

H. N. Ndi et al. (eds.), *Health Diplomacy in Africa*, Studies in Diplomacy and International Relations,
https://doi.org/10.1007/978-3-031-41249-3_10

the political correctness of different historical epochs. Here are some examples, beginning from the current and contemporary and going backwards in the history of their evolution: low- and middle-income countries (LMICs), least developed countries (LDCs)/low-income countries (LICs), low-resource settings, resource-poor countries, countries with limited resources, developing countries, underdeveloped countries, undeveloped countries, backward peoples, uncivilized peoples, uncultured peoples, barbarians, and savages.

At the dawn of colonization, epitomized in the Berlin Conference of 1884 (Craven, 2015), there was absolutely no problem referring to Africa as the "Dark Continent" and to Africans as savages, barbarians, and pagans. But when it became politically inappropriate to continue using such wild descriptions in the face of falsifying evidence, the colonialists cleverly evolved the terms to backward, uncivilized, and undeveloped peoples, and pretended to be in Africa on a civilizing mission. When even these evolved terms became uncomfortably jarring in the ears, it was time for their cleverness again to evolve and they invented underdeveloped and developing peoples and countries. From there they seamlessly moved to countries with limited resources, resource-poor countries, and low-resource settings. Currently, the politically correct expressions are LMICs and LICs.

All these colonial terms and concepts seek to throw a single blanket over very diverse peoples and countries for the convenience of their external colonizers and exploiters. There is nothing wrong with accurately descriptive terms like north Africa, south Africa, east Africa, west Africa, Africa north/south of the Sahara, etc., if used purely descriptively, but every part and every country of Africa is diverse and significantly different in many respects from the others. The communalities of Africans are in the historical, socio-cultural, and metaphysico-religious domains, in shared ideas, beliefs, experiences, and practices. But every African country or region ought to be called by its proper name as well as appreciated with all its specificities and not blanketed with others for the convenience of external colonizers and exploiters.

COVID-19 PANDEMIC AND THE WAR IN UKRAINE

Two global events, the COVID-19 pandemic and the War in Ukraine, have marked indelibly the history of the world in our epoch, the opening decades of the twenty-first century of the third millennium. These two events have impacted the continent of Africa as well as peoples of African descent all over the world in fundamentally troubling ways implying and occasioning a jolt in consciousness. The war in Ukraine, pitting Russia against the NATO is, for all intents and purposes, the third world war (WWIII) and this may not be evident simply because nuclear weapons have not yet been used as many people unconsciously expect for any WWIII. The war has reawakened Euro-Americans to doing what they know best how to do and this as far back in their history as one may want to investigate—warring. The war falls short only in the use of nuclear or atomic weapons but is veritably a world war involving all the superpowers of the world who are mobilizing all resources they can to ensure that the emerging new world order would be under their power and control. In that situation, as in the first (1914–1918) and second (1939–1945) world wars, Africa and Africans are victims, mercilessly exploited and manipulated by both sides of the conflict, each in its own rational self-interest. Thanks to the social media, this war has confirmed that Africa, Africans, people of African descent, and black people all over the world, for some unfathomable reason, are victims of deep-seated racial discrimination and persecution. In Ukraine during this war, we have witnessed African students, fleeing for safety like other human beings, discriminated against and denied war refugee entry into some European countries, in preference for cats and dogs.

Regarding COVID-19, it has clearly highlighted the fact that there is no part of world, including the African continent itself, where Africans are treated with equity vis-à-vis other human beings. Indifference is not permissible, let alone from Africans themselves, in the face of this situation. When the epidemic first erupted in 2019, the same procedures and attempted solutions—lockdown, social distancing, hand washing, mask wearing—applied in so-called developed countries, where the epidemic originated and has had its greatest casualties so far, had been prescribed if not completely applied in Africa and other parts of the so-called non-developed world by global health authorities, including triaging for scarce medical resources, with little consideration for contextual differences and specificities. For this reason, it was bemoaned in advance along with predictions of an on-coming catastrophe, that some African countries did not possess as much as a single respiratory medical ventilator. But what is any country where most people have no drinking water, where simple hygiene and sanitation leave everything to be desired, where the governing authorities seem never to have heard of primary healthcare, where the few modern hospitals that exist are places where health seekers go to die or to aggravate their health condition, if not contract new pathologies, what is a country of that description doing with medical ventilators? Moreover, God/Nature did not create human beings with the intention that they would need a ventilator for breathing at some point in their lives. Besides, in the so-called developed countries, where the number of medical ventilators is not so derisory, there was an acute shortage in the face of COVID-19, making triaging of patients in need of the ventilators necessary, giving rise to various theories of ethical triaging, a favourite intellectual sport or pastime and preoccupation of ethicists in the so-called developed world.

In the triaging business, Western ethicists, with only a few exceptions, seem for once to have achieved unanimity on one point: young people are to be prioritized over old people and those with a greater chance of living longer over those with less chance. This prioritization logic is very persuasive within a paradigm of economic utilitarian rationality, which rules the industrialized Western world. In my view, ethics must be based on indiscriminate respect for the environment, nature, and life, especially human life. All human beings simply as human beings, without any exceptions, are morally equal and equally valuable, from the first moment of their emergence into life to the last moment of their natural exit from life (Tangwa, 2007). To rationalize saving human lives or letting die based on personal individuating characteristics (race, age, complexion, size, sex, weight, height, etc.) appears to me ethically rather monstrously disquieting. Of course, no one can downplay the seriousness of the COVID-19 pandemic and the dilemmas it has created for healthcare systems around the world. And, with many existential quandaries, there is often no way of coming out without either doing or allowing harm to be done. This is one of many fundamental human limitations. However, this situation can be faced without writing a single prescription for all human societies, particularly without artificially categorizing moral equals based on ethically irrelevant criteria of discrimination, in the name of doing triage and doing so with a quiet conscience, if not a sense of moral uprightness.

The African continent was the last part of the globe to be reached by the COVID-19 epidemic. This tardiness led to speculative claims on social media that black people and people of African descent had a special immunity against the virus and that the predominantly hot temperatures in Africa were not conducive to propagation of the virus. The falsity of such claims was soon demonstrated when in Europe and America it became clear that the virus was particularly lethal for old people of all races and black people and African descendants of all ages.

In Africa the very first case of COVID-19 was reported in Egypt on 14 February 2020 (Aljazeera News, 2020), shortly before the World Health Organization (WHO) declared the epidemic a Public Health Emergency of International Concern (PHEIC) on 11 March 2020. By the time Lesotho recorded its first case on 13 May 2020, the epidemic had already answered present in all the 54 countries of Africa. In this situation, it soon became clear that the push of global health authorities in Africa was first and foremost for mass vaccinations of the populations with any of the experimental vaccines, when and if available, that the developed world had hurriedly manufactured. At bottom then, the interest of the so-called developed world in Africa in the face of the COVID-19 pandemic was first and foremost as a field of medical experimentation in the interest and benefit of global vaccine manufacturers and the governments which protect and profit from their highly profitable medically reckless ventures, including experimentation on human beings. Some people dispute the suggestion that some COVID-19 vaccines have been basically experimental vaccines. But the fact that they were hurriedly approved for use in humans and guaranteed neither protection from reinfection nor from infecting others and have required unforeseen boosters and even boosters to the boosters, clearly points to the fact that they were rushed to bypass pertinent medicine regulation. A Reuters report of 11 March 2020 talks of the resolution of a WHO meeting in February designed to coordinate a global response to the new coronavirus where scientists representing government-funded research organizations and drugmakers around the world agreed that the Covid-19 threat was so great that vaccine developers were encouraged to move quickly into human trials, even before animal testing was completed (Steenhuysen, 2020). Similarly, drug regulatory agencies in countries like the USA and UK granted temporary authorization to use vaccines like the Pfizer/BioNTech to MHRA in the period from 1 October to 2 December 2020, in the UK and Northern Ireland, but not for marketing purposes. The temporary nature of this authorization made the harmful effects of the aforementioned vaccines on humans unpredictable. (GOV.UK. 2023)

If after taking a vaccine and two boosters you are still susceptible to infection as well as to infecting others, and you don't know that you must be participating in open clinical experimentation, then I don't know what you do know.

Today it would clearly be stated upfront that taking the vaccine would not prevent reinfection or infecting others but that it would prevent severe illness and/or death. These, however, are facts that have been learned empirically after the introduction of the vaccine and not qualities that were known through rigorous tests before their deployment. And we must note the mutation in the very concept of a vaccine. In medical history, as we have known it, a vaccine is something taken to prevent an infection, not something taken to prevent severe illness and/or death.

CAMEROON, AN INTERESTING CASE STUDY

Cameroon would make a most interesting case study for COVID-19 on many counts. First, COVID-19 erupted and arrived in Africa while Cameroon has been engaged in a nasty civil war against the English-speaking minority, which is seeking separation and independence, based on a failed union organized by the United Nations in 1961 on behalf of the colonial powers of France and Great Britain (Cascais, 2021). Since 2017 when the war started, it has claimed about 5,000 innocent lives, displaced about 2 million people and destroyed about 500 villages (Longari, 2019). The Cameroon government is more interested in fighting and winning this war than in fighting COVID-19. Therefore, it turned a completely deaf ear to the call by the UN Secretary General for a cease-fire in the civil war, in the interest of fighting COVID-19 (Miller, 2020).

Secondly, with the first wave of COVID-19 infections in Cameroon in early March 2020 (CCOUSP Cameroon, 2020; Tih, 2020), the leader of the country, President Paul Biya, self-quarantined himself and completely disappeared from public space and was neither heard nor seen again until around mid-May 2020 when he was seen in a video with the French ambassador to Cameroon (Shaban, 2020) and subsequently briefly on 19 May, the eve of Cameroon's national day, on television making a brief speech. So, while the leaders of other countries were coming out personally almost daily to talk to their people and to give current statistics and instructions regarding COVID-19, all that was witnessed in Cameroon were Ministers claiming to have been instructed by the President to instruct the people to do this or that.

Thirdly, less than two weeks after imposing some half-hearted lockdown measure to contain the epidemic, the government, on the pretext of economic considerations, eased the lockdown measures, especially regarding the opening of bars, restaurants, and night clubs, and insisted only on mask wearing and hand washing. These measures, moreover, were not ensured or enforced in a serious manner, making the entire approach rather sloppy. Not surprisingly, infection cases somewhat escalated.

Fourthly, Cameroon, on the heels of Madagascar, came up with several plant-based remedies that seemed to cure COVID-19. In April 2020, Madagascar had officially launched a herbal medicine, COVID Organics (CVO), developed by the Malagasy Institute of Applied Research, from the Artemisia plant, well known for its anti-Malaria properties, which it claimed both prevents and cures COVID-19. Although the WHO was prompt in dismissing the claim that CVO cures COVID-19 and insisting that there is as yet no cure for the disease, other African countries were enthusiastic in placing orders for the medicine from Madagascar for their own COVID-19 patients and South Africa offered to carry out a confirmatory scientific analysis of the herbal mixture.

In Cameroon, there emerged a veritable plethora of plant-based cures for COVID-19 (Kindzeka, 2020; La Nouvelle Expression, 2020). Notable among these are the following:

1. A well-known traditional healer, Dr. Ngepah Julius, with more than twenty years of naturalistic practice, claims to have a cocktail, composed of a tea, a sirop, and a powder made from plants, that eliminates all the symptoms of COVID-19.

2. Another traditional healer, Mohamadoul Aminoudu, claims to have a plant-based remedy that he calls simply "Covid Cure" which is both curative and preventive, and of which he has distributed to date about 1,000 doses and cured about 400 COVID-19 cases.

3. Dr. Maurice Tazong's own herbal medicine against COVID-19 is called "Corovitaz", composed of vitamins, anti-bacteria, anti-parasites, and anti-inflamatories. He does not give an exact number but claims to have cured hundreds of COVID-19 patients.

4. In the case of Dr. Charles Hopson, he is a Cameroonian trained in Allopathic Western medicine in the USA where he runs a research laboratory "Doctor HOPSON Pharmaceuticals Labs" in collaboration with "Longevita Pharmaceuticals Laboratories". Dr. Hopson claims to have discovered a "magic cure" that he calls "Stop Corona" against COVID-19.

5. The last case here is that of the Catholic Archbishop of Douala, Mgr. Samuel Kleda, who announced the successful treatment of COVID-19 positive patients with a herbal mixture, "Elixir COVID"

and "Adsak COVID". The mixtures are administered free of charge at designated Catholic health centres upon presentation of a COVID-19 positive test result. So far, over 3,000 patients, among them some patients who were already on ventilators in state hospitals, have reportedly been successfully treated, including several medical doctors and health workers who had contracted the disease while handling the first wave of patients in the country.

Each of the above claimants of a cure for COVID-19 has reported about their remedy to the governmental authorities and on the media in the hope that it would be further investigated and officially approved. But, not surprisingly, the government as well as most medical scientists, is highly reticent if not dismissive of these claims, preferring to wait for instructions or cues from the so-called International Community and the WHO. Governments and Western-educated elite of all African countries urgently need mental decolonization (Wa Thiong'o, 1992; Wiredu, 1997). Their life and well-being are parasitical to exploitative colonialism and neo-colonialism in their own countries. If science is evidence-based, then the scientific merit of these herbal medicines (why do they work and what is it in each of them that makes it work?) cannot lightly be brushed aside but ought to be investigated with rigor and in all scientific objectivity.

Objectivity, of course, must not be confined to a particular paradigm or practice where procedures carried out outside of own laboratories and control are not qualify-able as objective; that would be subjective-objectivity. The scientific and medical merit of efficacious herbal remedies ought to be investigated and in fact ought to form the main focus of the country's efforts in the face of COVID-19. Cameroon is remarkable for its biodiversity—plant, animal, and human—and most of its inhabitants still live close to nature; and this plethora of possible cures is a fruit of that biodiversity and a relatively natural mode of living. This is a very good thing for Cameroon which, otherwise, presents perhaps the worst global case scenario for tackling COVID-19.

AFRICA AND THE WORLD HEALTH ORGANIZATION

The WHO is perhaps the most important agency of the United Nations with a global mandate whose importance is evident and acknowledged by all and sundry. All around the world, governments, especially ministries of public health, healthcare providers, and medical researchers, listen to the

WHO and sometimes obey its recommendations without questions, like dummies. For these reasons, the WHO needs to be not only highly professional in its actions and pronouncements but also transparently fair to all the different global communities and competing interests in global health in their variegated diversities and differences. Unfortunately, the WHO seems not yet anything of the sort (Tangwa and Afolabi, 2019). Whenever the WHO declares that there is no treatment for a disease, what it clearly seems to mean is that there is no drug approved by the US Food and Drug Administration (FDA) or duly licensed in any part of the industrialized developed world. For an organization with a global mandate, this is not good enough except on the assumption that Globalization is no more and no less than Westernization (Tangwa, 1999). Furthermore, the WHO seems to be under the subtle influence and control of for-profit medical research with a clear preference for research on vaccines on account of their high economic profitability, since a vaccine is prescribed for everybody, ill or not ill. In Africa, the WHO has conducted or facilitated the conduct of ethically questionable vaccine research such as in the case of Ebola in Guinea and the Democratic Republic of the Congo (Cohen, 2014; Tangwa et al., 2018).

There is a strong lobby for COVID-19 vaccination even though the vaccines available are evidently experimental, requiring repeated shots and continuous boosters based on their actions and observed efficacity in the face of a continuously mutating virus. In Africa, this lobby has taken the contours of a campaign, given vaccine hesitancy and the fact that it is coming at a time many people, thanks to the social media and to so-called conspiracy theories, are getting to hear for the first time about the possible disadvantages or dangers of vaccines. Vaccine development generally takes several years if not decades, but COVID-19 vaccine development seems to have been on a super-fast track. And with COVID-19, the WHO had already articulated "criteria for ethical acceptability" of human challenge studies (Jamrozik et al., 2021)—deliberate infection of a healthy individual with a virus for any candidate vaccine against COVID-19.

Proponents and defenders of COVID-19 vaccines testing in Africa are, arguably, mostly eminent scientists and scientific projects managers/coordinators. The gist of the recurring thrust of their several arguments for vaccine testing is that Africa bears 25 per cent of the global burden of disease but conducts only 2 per cent of clinical trials; that Africa's virtual absence from the "clinical trials map" is a big problem; that it is vital for Africans to take part in vaccine trials or else the aim of finding a vaccine that works worldwide and not just for the richer nations would be jeopardized; that Africa risks being 'locked out' from the world to continue in its legacy of exclusion, inequality, and poverty; that different circumstances and genetic profiles affect how a vaccine may work and Africa needs to take part in vaccine tests to ensure having a vaccine that works in Africa. These are well-resourced arguments by those who evidently have a vested stake in the vaccine they envisage being tested in Africa and they therefore sound a little desperate like planned project drives, if not rehearsed propaganda. A detail in these arguments is worth further consideration. If genetic makeup and circumstances are so important for a vaccine, that would seem to be a very good reason why the richer developed countries, that share the same worldview and underpinning culture, with a similar level of material affluence should develop their own vaccine while people in Africa and other different regions, who share a common culture and worldview, should also develop theirs. And when were the vaccines currently being administered in Africa tested against African genetic profiles to make sure that they are suitable and workable in the context?

DIFFERENT HEALTHCARE SYSTEMS

There needs to be different healthcare systems around the globe, each harmonized with its environment, instead of the current situation where the healthcare system of the industrialized developed world has been globalized as a consequence of colonialism, domination, and exploitation and imposed in different parts of the world. The current dilemmas of rationing in the face of COVID-19 as well as the challenges of vaccine development are highly accentuated because of a system in which healthcare is inextricably dovetailed with commerce, for profit procedures and attendant morally blind forces (Callahan and Wasunna, 2006). There is a need to question whether the institutions and traditions of medicine and healthcare, developed from Hippocratic traditions, as they have been known in the Western world, are morally compatible with market thinking, theory, and practice? There seems to be such an intrusive conflict of values between medicine and the market that they should not be joined no matter how attractive the apparent consequences appear to be. But this important consideration evidently seems to have been overtaken by the sheer evolution and momentum of things. In short, it seems that liberal capitalist economic thinking and mindset has overwhelmed everything else in the

Western world and is in the process of overwhelming the rest of the world through colonization and globalization.

In pre-colonial traditional Africa (at least in most parts of it) medicine and the art of healing were completely divorced from the market (involving sale and/or exchange of goods and services) (Tangwa, 2010). The idea of paying for treatment, medicine, healthcare, etc., is largely a legacy of colonialism and its introduction of a monetarized economy and Allopathic Western-style medicine in Africa. Ever since, market practices have become increasingly important in the medicine and healthcare domain, engulfing even traditional medicine, as a consequence of which many quacks and charlatans have invaded the latter. There are three main arms in present-day healthcare delivery systems in sub-Saharan Africa north of the Limpopo, particularly in West and Central Africa, with which I am directly relatively familiar: (a) uncorrupted traditional medicine which operates mainly in the rural areas and has been receding into history, (b) modern Allopathic Western-style medicine which operates through hospitals and pharmacies, and (c) medicinal hawkers who try to combine traditional medicine with modern medicine attitudes and practices and who operate mostly in urban areas.

One of the glaring scandals of the "medicine-market" system is the 'devaluation' of old people in the Western world, forgetting that some of these old people are directly or indirectly responsible for the 'successes' of the very system and that everybody without exception naturally tends towards becoming old while death remains one of those events in every human life that cannot accurately be foreseen. By the way, within another paradigm and imaginable system different from this dominant Western one, I know that older people, in situations of scarcity requiring rationing, would be the first ones to opt out of receiving treatment in the interest of their own offspring and younger folk of their communities.

African culture seems to have stumbled on a satisfactory manner of, for example, balancing the needs and interests of older people and those of younger people in the society. The main problem with ageing after the peak of youthfulness is the progressive loss of physical and mental energy culminating in a situation where the old person becomes once again like the helpless baby s/he was after first emergence into the world. At that stage, the old person could easily become helplessly lonely and depressed. Traditional African culture addresses this situation by apportioning progressive privileges, honours, and respect the older one grows. Most of these, like bowing, genuflecting, or prostrating while greeting an older person, carrying out an errand from an older person always on the run, ceremonially always offering, say, the gizzard of a chicken prepared for a meal to the oldest person in the household, etc., are completely empty of what may be called "cash value" but are psychologically very satisfying. For that reason, people within African cultures can face the process of ageing without much anxiety but rather by looking forward to attendant privileges which they can flaunt in the face of younger people who need not bother anyway, as they also can look forward to the same privileges in due course. Above all, the African communal style of living is fundamentally subversive of individualism, aloneness, and loneliness.

I don't have any prescription on how to do triage in the face of scarcity in a difficult situation like the COVID-19 pandemic. Several plausible suggestions are available (Archard & Caplan, 2020; Emanuel et al., 2020; NASEM, 2020; Singh & Moodley, 2020). However, medical personnel, given their well-known moral sensibility and sensitivity, their Hippocratic traditions, even professional oaths, should not confuse economic considerations and quandaries with ethics or be waiting for outsiders, even those wearing the costume of globality, to tell them how to resolve dilemmas in their own work at a critical moment in human survival history. In any event, it is evident that one's personal immune system, harmonized with one's environment, the food one eats and one's habitual activities, is the best and most powerful mechanism for fighting all diseases including epidemic diseases and ill-health in general. The immune system can be strengthened or supported but, if it breaks down irremediably, death is accurately signalled even if some artificial means are found to prolong some living functions of the body for a while. Any healthcare system ought to take this fact into serious consideration.

It is odd that many African countries, without basic hygiene and sanitation, without any primary healthcare system, without even a glance at their own traditional healthcare systems and the values on which over 80 per cent of their populations depend, focus their attention and public resources on imitative high-tech medicine developed elsewhere and not yet domesticated on African soil. High-tech medicine is a patent of the industrialized developed world, harmonized with its general culture and traditional medicine from which it evolved, and those outside of that world cannot fully participate in it except as colonized, dependent, subjugated, and exploited people. The imperative alternative is to acquire and use science and technology to modernize their traditional medicine and, if need be, to develop it to high-tech medicine. Otherwise, the best that is achievable is what is observable, namely, that the beneficiaries of high-tech medicine in Africa and the rest of the so-called developing world, (developing to where?), are the small percentage of Western-educated elite who, since colonization, have connived with the colonizers to aid and facilitate the subjugation and exploitation of their own lands and people in exchange for comfortable careers that permit a developed world lifestyle in the developing world and, above all, power and authority without any responsibility. These are the happy slaves of the dominated and dependent African system. This situation needs to change now.

MENTAL DECOLONIZATION

Africans need serious mental decolonization (Wiredu & Oladipo, 1995). The current ruling groups in Africa are generally the second generation of those colonized Africans who benefited from a modernized education based on literacy as a corollary of colonization. In the era of their immediate predecessors, the pioneers of modern formal education in Africa, they used to be evaluated by being asked such questions as: "*when* and by *whom* was the River Niger discovered?" Those who readily answered "1796 by Mungo Park" were rated the most intelligent pupils, who later made it to Oxford, Cambridge, Harvard, Yale, etc. Those who were paralysed into silence by the oddity and strangeness of such a question were the dull ones who never made it to anywhere. Those who "made it" came back with "the golden fleece" and took over the reins of governance from the colonial masters now that the latter had decided to grant "independences" all over the continent.

Accessing power and staying on in power seems such a desperate thing for the inheritors of colonial power in Africa. Many of these inheritors of power and authority without any responsibility, without any internal checks and balances, are contracted to protect the interests of the erstwhile colonial master or external manipulator in any case and, for the rest, they can do just what they like as leaders, including eliminating any opponents or threats to their power and authority, converting public resources into private property and handing over power and authority when they are done or gone to their offspring. These admittedly strong claims are easily verifiable, especially in what are called "Francophone" countries in Africa. That is why the continent is in such an incredibly despicable mess, despite abundant resources, both material and human. Decolonization and good governance are the greatest needs of the continent now, without which nothing else is likely to go right. Africans need to go into the process of learning and relearning many things and one of these is the recognition of the illusion which makes them see well-being and prosperity only overseas across the ocean or the Sahara Desert. The illusion is symbolically circumscribed by the futility of searching far and wide in vain for something hidden in one's own pocket.

DECOLONIZATION AND DEVELOPMENT

Now, Africa needs decolonization more urgently than a vaccine against COVID-19; and that is not to minimize the importance or urgent necessity of a COVID-19 vaccine (Tangwa, 2021). The partition of Africa in 1884 at Berlin by European imperial nations marked one of the greatest crimes against humanity in human history, in that it considered a whole continent including its human occupants and resources simply as economic assets for the technologically more advanced peoples. Ever since, the world has witnessed many subterfuges at redressing the situation, from granting of 'independencies' through 'structural adjustment' programmes to 'development' grants and loans. These are matters of global justice and fairness. As an educated African and a Cameroonian, it is with a sense of embarrassment bordering on shame that I learned only as recently as 2018, thanks to social media, that Cameroon, like many other French-speaking countries of the continent, had signed a pact with the colonial master, France, in the couple of years preceding so-called granting of independence, to the effect that all the resources in the country underground belong to France and that France was also in charge of the educational system at all levels. It is time for Africa to assume and assert its total decolonization/independence and the impact of COVID-19 offers as good an occasion and opportunity as it has ever had to do by starting again from the scratch, as it were.

RESEARCH AND DEVELOPMENT

Research and development are closely connected. Research is the greatest enabler of development, and no country can develop without engaging in fundamental research and utilizing its results as an evidential base for its developmental policies and projects. The greatest impediment to development in Africa is the fact that governmental authorities do not seem to realize sufficiently the importance of research for development with the consequence that research is not adequately funded, if at all, leaving all manner of foreign explorers and adventurers to invade the continent as funders of research of dubious value to the continent and its peoples.

As a matter of fact, many tertiary institutions, universities, and research laboratories in Africa rely extensively on external funding from the industrialized developed world for any research they carry out. This situation has the important shortcoming that most of the research carried out in Africa is externally conceptualized and blueprinted and, consequently, scarcely addresses the real needs of the local situation or the priorities logically dictated by the existential pressures of the context. Besides, external funders of research, even if they are completely altruistic in their intentions, have a conception of the world and of development that is, at best, different from, if not antithetical to, a proper and anchored conception of development in the African context. An example from the healthcare domain is the recent reckless release of genetically modified mosquitoes in Burkina Faso under the pretext of carrying out research on malaria. Mosquitoes need no visas to travel and the risks to which the government of that country irresponsibly has exposed its environment and citizens by authorizing the reckless release are now the risks of the entire continent.

Proper and sustainable development in Africa needs to take into full account the fact that it is a previously colonized continent not yet convincingly decolonized. Moreover, development in Africa must move in the opposite direction from the European conception which envisages development through imitation of its own model, involving progressive industrialization, urbanization, and globalization. Urbanization has been a disaster in Africa, resulting in heavy and irrational rural-urban migration, complete breakdown in the traditional African worldview, mores, and behaviours. Rubbish dumps called cities in Africa, without proper roads or parking spaces, full of motorcycles, second-hand cars, and trucks, which render moving around a nightmare, have rapidly grown in Africa in the post-colonial period.

In pre-colonial Africa, the villages (where the balance between human beings, non-human animals, plants, and nature is sustained) were the centres of the diverse cultures and way of life of the people. Any genuine and sustainable development in Africa needs to begin from its villages. A carefully conceptualized policy of *villagization* rather than *urbanization* is what will be able to lead to genuine and sustainable development in Africa; otherwise, we will continue to witness countries where a small proportion of the people gets incredibly rich both at home and abroad on public resources, while the vast majority remain under an illusion which propels many of them to risk limb and life migrating to other countries where they can earn a decent living doing jobs that are only a shouting distance from slave labour.

CONCLUSION

COVID-19 is one of the most devastating epidemics in human history. It has affected all continents of the world, all countries, and all human communities although in different ways and to varying degrees, thereby truly earning the title of a pandemic. The war in Ukraine that has broken out in course of this pandemic is a veritable world war pitting Russia against NATO and drawing all the world's superpowers into the conflict. Different peoples in different parts of the world who survive both the epidemic and the war must learn what lessons they can learn from the two events to move forward with their lives.

The racism against Africans, black people, and people of African descent that has independently accompanied COVID-19 (HRW, 2020) as well as the on-going world war in nearly all parts of the world (especially in the USA, Europe, and China) indicates that the lessons to be learned from these events by the African continent, Africans, and people of African descent all over the world, are not only important but also urgent. Foremost amongst these lessons is the urgent imperative of decolonizing healthcare in Africa.

Africa is the least developed of the continents and has been a colonized and exploited continent for several centuries. In the face of COVID-19 and the Ukraine war, Africa has been looked upon mainly as the continent where vaccine tests can speedily and cost-effectively be carried out or support and resources secured, for the benefit of the rest of the world. The enthusiasts for testing virus vaccines in Africa, conceived, and developed elsewhere, including many Africans whose gaze is fixated on benefactors in the rich developed world who ensure for them a comfortable career and a developed world lifestyle in the developing world, have all characteristically ignored or downplayed the remarkable simple treatments of diseases in several African countries with plant-based medicines, the very source of the sophisticated synthetic medicines of the Allopathic pharmaceutical industry that are so unaffordable even if available to the populations of Africa. When anyone, not excluding vaccinologists, falls ill with a contagious life-threatening epidemic disease, the first and most logical thing to do is urgently to try saving life by looking for a remedy to the illness, not to research for a vaccine for future protection against the illness. Vaccines should be carefully developed outside of emergency health situations.

This situation is teaching a powerful course whose first lesson is that Africa at this moment in its history more urgently needs decolonization than anything else (Fofana, 2021). Such decolonization is the condition for developing medicines and vaccines that address the real health problems of the continent without external imposition and exploitation. Genuine decolonization should be followed by transforming the continent into a place where all black people and all people of African descent can feel completely at home; where all human beings, no matter from where they are coming, can feel at home because of the pervasive spirit and practice of Ubuntu (Tangwa, 2019). Only in this way will there be an eventual paradigm shift in the rest of the world, where Africans, black people, and people of African descent everywhere around the globe, might be regarded and treated as human beings with moral equality and equity with all other human beings.

REFERENCES

Aljazeera News. (2020, May 26). Egypt confirms coronavirus case, the first in Africa. https://www.aljazeera.com/news/2020/02/egypt-confirms-coronavirus-case-africa-200214190840134.html.

Archard, D., & Caplan, A. (2020). Is it wrong to prioritise younger patients with covid-19? *British Medical Journal, 369*. https://doi.org/10.1136/bmj.m1509

Callahan, D., & Wasunna, A. (2006). *Medicine and the market: Equity v.* Johns Hopkins University Press.

Cascais, A. (2021). 5 years of violent civil war in Cameroon. Deutsche Welle (DW). https://www.dw.com/en/separatism-in-cameroon-5-years-of-violent-civil-war/a-59369417.

CCOUSP Cameroon. (2020). Rapport Situation Covid-19 Cameroun N°12., Centre de Coordination des Opérations d'Urgences de Santé Publique: 6. https://www.ccousp.cm/download/rapport-situation-covid-19-cameroun-n12/

Cohen, J. (2014). Ebola vaccine: Little and late. *Science, 345*(6203), 1441. https://doi.org/10.1126/science.345.6203.1441

Craven, M. (2015). Between law and history: The Berlin Conference of 1884–1885 and the logic of free trade. *London Review of International Law, 3*(1), 31–59. https://doi.org/10.1093/lril/lrv002

Emanuel, E. J., Persad, R., Upshur, B., Thome, M., Parker, A., Glickman, C., Zhang, C., Boyle, M., & Smith & Phillips J. P. (2020). Fair allocation of scarce medical resources in the time of Covid-19. *New England Journal of Medicine, 382*(21), 2049–2055. https://doi.org/10.1056/nejmsb2005114

Fofana, M. O. (2021). Decolonising global health in the time of COVID-19. *Global Public Health, 16*(8–9), 1155–1166. https://doi.org/10.108 0/17441692.2020.1864754

GOV.UK. (March 2023). Vaccine BNT162b2—Conditions of authorisation under Regulation 174—2 December 2020, amended on 30 December 2020, 28 January 2021, 30 March 2021, 19 May 2021, 04 June 2021, 29 July 2021, 9 September 2021, 27 September. https://www.gov.uk/government/publi-cations/regulatory-approval-of-pfizer-biontech-vaccine-for-covid-19/conditions-of-authorisation-for-pfizerbiontech-covid-19-vaccine

HRW. (2020, May 26). China: Covid-19 discrimination against Africans-forced quarantines, evictions, refused services in Guangzhou. https://www.hrw.org/news/2020/05/05/china-covid-19-discrimination-against-africans

Jamrozik, E., Littler, K., Bull, S., Emerson, C., Kang, G., Kapulu, M., Rey, E., Saenz, C., Shah, S., Smith, P. G., Upshur, R., Weijer, C., & Selgelid, M. J. (2021). Key criteria for the ethical acceptability of COVID-19 human challenge studies: Report of a WHO Working Group. *Vaccine, 39*(4), 633–640. https://apps.who.int/iris/handle/10665/331976

Kindzeka, M. E. (2020, May 02). Hundreds rush for popular cleric's herbal COVID 'Cure' in Cameroon. https://www.voanews.com/a/covid-19-pandemic_hundreds-rush-popular-clerics-herbal-covid-cure-cameroon/6188607.html.

La Nouvelle Expression. (2020, June 9). Traitement du coronavirus: les solutions camerounaises font-elles peur. n° 5234. *Actu Cameroun.* https://actucamer-oun.com/2020/06/09/traitement-du-coronavirus-les-solutions-camerounaises-font-elles-peur/.

Longari, M. (2019, November 9). Cameroon's president vows 'national dialogue' to ease tensions with anglophone separatists. *France 24.* https://www.france24.com/en/20190911-cameroonian-president-biya-national-dialogue-anglophone-separatists.

Miller, A. (2020, May 13). Call unanswered: A review of responses to the UN appeal for a global ceasefire. *ACLED.* https://acleddata.com/2020/05/13/call-unanswered-un-appeal/.

NASEM. (2020). Ensuring equity in COVID-19 vaccine allocation globally. In B. Kahn, L. Brown, W. Foege, & H. Gayle (Eds.), *Framework for equitable allocation of COVID-19 vaccine.* National Academies Press. https://www.ncbi.nlm.nih.gov/books/NBK564100/

Shaban, A. A. (2020, April 17). Cameroon's 'missing president' reappears, holds COVID-19 meeting. *Africa News.* https://www.africanews.com/2020/04/17/cameroon-s-missing-president-reappears-holds-covid-19-meeting//.

Singh, J. A., & Moodley, K. (2020). Critical care triaging in the shadow of COVID-19: Ethics considerations. *South African Medical Journal, 110*(5), 355–359. https://doi.org/10.7196/SAMJ.2020.v110i5.14778

Steenhuysen, J. (2020, March 11). As pressure for coronavirus vaccine mounts, scientists debate risks of accelerated testing. https://www.reuters.com/article/us-health-coronavirus-vaccines-insight-idUSKBN20Y1GZ.

Tangwa, G. (1999). Globalisation or Westernisation? ethical concerns in the whole bio-business. *Bioethics, 13*(3–4), 218–226. https://doi.org/10.1111/1467-8519.00149

Tangwa, G. B. (2007). Moral status of embryonic stem cells: Perspective of an African villager. *Bioethics, 21*(8), 449–457. https://doi.org/10.1111/j.1467-8519.2007.00582.x

Tangwa, G. B. (2010). *Elements of African Bioethics in a Western Frame*. Langaa Research & Publishing.

Tangwa, G. B. (2019). Bioethics and Ubuntu, The transformative global potential of an African concept. In H. Lauer & H. Yitah (Eds.), *The tenacity of truthfulness: Philosophical essays in honour of Mogobe Bernard Ramose* (pp. 239–249). EARS Publishing Company.

Tangwa, G. B. (2021). Covid-19, the WHO, and the apparent collapse of traditional medical research ethics. *Indian Journal of Medical Ethics, 6*(2), 1–12. https://doi.org/10.20529/ijme.2021.028

Tangwa, G. B., & Afolabi, M. O. (2019). Global emerging pathogens and the (prescriptive) role of the World Health Organization. In G. Tangwa, A. Abayomi, S. Ujewe, & N. Munung (Eds.), *Socio-cultural dimensions of emerging infectious diseases in Africa*. Springer. https://doi.org/10.1007/978-3-030-17474-3_10

Tangwa, G. B., Browne, K., & Schroeder, D. (2018). Ebola vaccine trials. In D. Schroeder, J. Cook, F. Hirsch, S. Fenet, & V. Muthuswamy (Eds.), *Ethics dumping: Case studies from north-south research collaborations*. Springer International Publishing. https://library.oapen.org/bitstream/id/ceee0ec0-e484-4626-8907-8e0a34e07847/1002193.pdf

Tih, F. (2020, March 06). Cameroon confirms first coronavirus case. https://www.aa.com.tr/en/africa/cameroon-confirms-first-coronavirus-case/1756866.

Wa Thiong'o, N. (1992). *Decolonising the mind: The politics of language in African literature*. East African Publishers.

Wiredu, K. (1997). The need for conceptual decolonization in African philosophy. In F. Wimmeer (Ed.), *H. Kimmerle* (pp. 11–22). *Philosophy and democracy in intercultural Perspective/Philosophie et démocratie en perspective interculturelle*. https://brill.com/display/title/30704

Wiredu, K., & Oladipo, O. (1995). *Conceptual decolonization in African philosophy: Four essays*. Hope Publications.

CHAPTER 11

Conclusion

Humphrey Ngala Ndi

Most of the contributors to this book think that African governments and the African Union, the continent's multilateral diplomatic platform, can only sustainably address health and other problems on the African continent by committing African resources to them, rather than always adopting the fashionable posture of looking elsewhere for help all the time. It is said, if you do not do small things right, you will never be able to do big things right. If African governments can enhance good public governance through an equitable justice system, a lot of resources which would have been mismanaged or misappropriated will become available for development projects on the continent.

Unfortunately, as rich as the continent is known to be, in terms of its natural resources and a youthful population, it is paradoxically classified as the poorest place in the world. Poverty in Africa cannot be eradicated through borrowing and aid. The roots of the continent's poverty are related to the system of colonial exploitation which has persisted up to the post-colonial period, albeit more subtle but very determined. Consequently,

H. N. Ndi (✉)
High Commission for the Republic of Cameroon in London, London, UK

University of Yaounde I, Yaounde, Cameroon

© The Author(s), under exclusive license to Springer Nature Switzerland AG 2023
H. N. Ndi et al. (eds.), *Health Diplomacy in Africa*, Studies in Diplomacy and International Relations,
https://doi.org/10.1007/978-3-031-41249-3_11

225

the continent earns comparatively very little from its reliance on primary commodities in international trade where prices are subject to change ever so often. Sadly, the structures of most of the continent's economies are still dominated by primary activities. Though some pundits blame this condition on external factors and the nature of the unequal relationship Africa entertains with the advanced countries of Europe, Asia, and North America, we think that the causes of underdevelopment are inherent in the nature of the post-colonial African polity created and fashioned by the colonists rather as spaces of economic exploitation, than political and national harmony. That has profoundly affected national cohesion and enforced strong centrifugal tendencies on a continent where the populations of various states display very diverse ethnic, cultural, historical, and language characteristics. Ethnic diversity within African states has remained the most negatively exploited characteristic of the continent by outsiders whose interest is in keeping it weak to facilitate exploitation, and African politicians who use it for political or military leverage as they seek power.

Political power that relies on ethnic mobilisation inevitably breeds nepotism, incompetence and injustice, the seeds of resistance, insurrections, and violence reminiscent of collapsed or failed states. Countries undergoing violence or civil wars are often described as failed states because their governments have lost control over the territory, economy, or population and are unable to provide basic security services and governance in general. In 2022, the Fragile States Index, formerly known as the Failed States Index, classified 54 countries in the world in one of the following categories of fragility (economic, political, and social): very high alert, high alert, alert, and high warning. Thirty-seven of these countries were in Africa. In their over sixty years of self-rule, few countries in Africa have not experienced such failure.

This narration is not unconnected to the subject of this book as may be perceived remotely. However, without strong and stable legitimate governments all over Africa, the AU, a most cherished continental ideal unanimously ratified by African leaders in Lomé in 2000, will never achieve its goals. The strength of the AU directly lies on its members. It is thus, naïve to think that a country facing internal disintegration (economic decline, human flight and brain drain, uneven development, weak state legitimacy, poor public services, poor human rights and lawlessness, demographic pressures, external intervention, and pressures from refugees and internally displaced person…) will commit fully to the organisation. It will normally commit more to tackling its existential threats than supporting the AU. In other words, without strong sovereign states in Africa, there will be no hope of a strong AU.

That said, we think that if the AU must achieve the 2063 vision of an integrated, prosperous, and peaceful Africa, a strongly proactive stands against bad governance must become its priority. It must not be voluntary like the African Peer Review Mechanism to which only a few willing countries subscribed but must be used as a compulsory standard for adherence to the organisation with risks of sanctions including even suspension or expulsion in the case of non-compliance. This is so because, we believe that legitimate and just governments are a cure for many of Africa's woes. When Africans shall come to a point in time where they are able to freely participate democratically in the governance of their polities, most of their fragilities will retreat in favour of the emergence of a truly national feeling and identity in most countries.

Without the emergence of strongly legitimate states in Africa, all the resources deployed by the AU to foster intra-African cooperation are a waste. If ordinary Africans cannot connect with each other confidently and freely; if the freedom of movements of people and goods remains rhetorical; and if inter-state diplomacy remains an elitist project; the AU would have failed to meet the continent's objectives even before it started.

The expression 'if you want to go fast, go alone, if you want to go far go together', though of an unknown origin, bears the same conceptual meaning as *unbuntu*, the Zulu word which means 'I am what I am because of who we all are'. In principle, that is the foundation of multilateralism which has dominated the world for over a century today, starting with the founding of the League of Nations in 1919, and replaced by the United Nations in 1945. All continental regions in the world have organised their countries into some economic and political unions—Association of Southeast Asian Nations, the European Union, the North American Free Trade Agreement, Mercosur, and the African Union, among others. These speak to the perceived mutual benefits of collective endeavours where the benefits of growth and development are shared across countries of different levels of progress and achievement with inbuilt levelling-up mechanisms. Notwithstanding, benefits accruing to such organisations created on the ashes of the colonial enterprise like the Commonwealth of Nations and *La Francophonie* disproportionately favour the former colonising powers. This is evident in the unequal balance of power between the UK and the rest of the members of the Commonwealth as the organisation is headquartered in London and the English sovereign, its natural head. It is the same with *La Francophonie*, which though headed by an elected Secretary-General is also headquartered in Paris. This has also given France a vantage positions over other members in the organisation. Through these organisations, these countries continue to exert substantial influences over their former colonial possessions, through arrangements which fall under public diplomacy, international development, global health, and development aid. These skewed relationships exacerbate domination, subservience, and the dependency of African states on their former colonial masters. Economic, social, and political dependency has been the hallmark of the African continent since the end of imperialism.

Early African politicians who led most of the continent into independence between the 1950s and the 1970s were unable to conduct such reforms in education as would have severed the umbilical cord with Europe and charted a new development path for the continent. By maintaining and reinforcing the European model, in form and content, the training of the continent's leaders (teachers, scientists, jurists, diplomats, administrators…) strengthened this dependency as the post-colonial African school system became even more European. Coloniality and the dependency of the African mind is an evident feature of Africa today underscoring the deep impact of colonial subjugation on the African psychic. As African countries continue to entertain intricate economic and political relationships with Europe, less attention is devoted to intra-African cooperation. Many AU member states share their loyalties between the AU and their former colonisers with whom aid for trade arrangements exist. That may explain why some African countries were fast to sign and start the implementation of the Economic Partnership Agreements (EPA) with the European Union, a trade-for-aid arrangement, and may be lukewarm towards the Africa Continental Free Trade Area (ACFTA), as no aid enticements are involved. Similarly, some African leaders will rush to attend a US-Africa Summit, China-Africa Summit, and the Tokyo International Conference of African Development (TICAD) than they would an AU Summit.

That is one of the main reasons why the organisation cannot even stand on its feet financially as many members only reluctantly contribute to its coffers. It has failed to unite Africans around its ideals, and it is a scandal for African leaders to allow the wheels of a pan-African organisation like the AU to be greased by foreign rational state actors like China, Japan, France, and many others in that category. No doubt, the first response by the AU to emergencies on the continent is to call on the support of its external partners, not even AU members.

Added to weak financial commitment is the fact that few African countries are spared violent conflict caused by depraved governments that derive their power not from popular consensus, but from the creepy influences and corrupt activities of multinational corporations in connivance with local elites especially in resource-rich countries. Multilateral corporations representing foreign capital have been known to meddle in political processes in resource-rich countries where they lobby by secretly financing the powers bids of politicians, they think will protect their business interests against the potentially uncooperative and stiff-lip ones. Politicians who succumb to such lobbyists soon realise they must deliver social and economic development to their people as well as provide favourable investment incentives to the foreign multinationals. In this dilemma, the interest of the people has often been sacrificed for the multinational investors. The cases of the Democratic Republic of the Congo (DRC) whose mineral wealth is coveted by world leading industrial nations is a palpable illustration and needs no further elucidation.

Notwithstanding this plethora of negative energy on the continent, the AU has made remarkable strides albeit in planning the development of the continent in all sectors encapsulated in Agenda 2063 though the question of the sources of funding to achieve it still begs for a convincing answer (African Union Commission, 2015).

It is thus evident from the foregone paragraphs that political commitment and financing are key issues in Africa's path to economic and social development including health. For the institutional arrangements of health diplomacy on the continent to succeed, a few obvious recommendations must be implemented.

- Borrowing from the German-British statistician, Ernst Friedrich Schumacher in his book 'Small is Beautiful', 'an ounce of practice is generally more than a ton of theory, the AU needs a new orientation of its approach based on practice and not theory (Schumacher, 1973). Planning instruments like the Lagos Plan of Action (1980); the Abuja Declaration on health financing (2001); and the African Continental Free Trade Association (2012) have remained on paper, yet more policy instruments are crafted and ratified by member states every time. If the policies mentioned above are not implemented over the years as designed, how will Africans look up to the AU for the success of Agenda 2063? Perhaps one of the problems with such policies is the customary trend to count on external donors for implementation. If the AU and its implementing agencies like the Africa CDC, the Africa Medicine Association, the Partnership for African Vaccine Manufacturing, must achieve their objectives, it must learn to depend first on its own resources and home-grown solutions to African problems as a means of building its own capacity over the traditionally exogenous solutions its leaders have for so long been accustomed to. The non-state actors notably African diaspora communities have proven to be invaluable partners in Africa's development and should be useful here if recognised and wooed rather than suspected and despised as has been the case with some African states.

- Research into the potentially enormous pharmacological wealth of African ecosystems will need to be intensified by African scientists with the active backing of policy makers at the AU and different ministries of health. By so doing, pharmaceutical inventions may be patented to African scientists and the African Medicine Agency as a continental regulatory agency with the responsibility to approve medicines invented in Africa, for the use of Africans like the Food and Drug Administration (FDA) in the USA; the Medicines and Healthcare Products Regulatory Agency (MHRA) in the UK; the National Medical Products Administration (NMPA) in China; and the Central Drugs Standards Control Organisation (CDSCO) in India among many others. This will be an imperative stage in decolonising medical practice in Africa.

- The African Union Assembly must be courageous to sanction countries which do not contribute regularly to its coffers and the African Peer Review Mechanism set up by New Partnership for Africa's Development (NEPAD) in 2003 as a voluntary self-monitor for governance and performance should be reformed and placed under the African Union Commission, to monitor, and report to the AU Assembly on democratic and political, economic, and corporate governance. In turn, this organ will help, reprimand, or even sanction governments which are underperforming. This may reduce the frequency of violent conflict on the continent.

REFERENCES

Africa Union Commission. (2015). Agenda 2063: The Africa we want. https://au.int/sites/default/files/documents/36204-doc-agenda2063_popular_version_en.pdf

Schumacher, E. F. (1973). *Small is beautiful: Economics as if people mattered.* HarperPerennial.

INDEX

© The Author(s), under exclusive license to Springer Nature Switzerland AG 2023
H. N. Ndi et al. (eds.), *Health Diplomacy in Africa*, Studies in Diplomacy and International Relations,
https://doi.org/10.1007/978-3-031-41249-3

Printed and bound by CPI Group (UK) Ltd, Croydon, CR0 4YY

11/12/2024

01804248-0001